Protect Your Prostate

Dr. Michael Colgan

For The First Time, The World-Renowned Colgan Institute Reveals Its Program For A Healthy Prostate

www.applepublishing.com

*The Information contained in this book was prepared from medical and scientific sources which are referenced herein and are believed to be accurate and reliable. However, the opinions expressed herein by the author do not necessarily represent the opinions or the views of the publisher. Nor should the information herein be used to treat or to prevent any medical condition unless it is used with the full knowledge, compliance and agreement of your personal physician or other licensed health care professional. Readers are strongly advised to seek the advice of their personal health care professional(s) before proceeding with **any** changes in **any** health care program.*

FIRST EDITION

Canadian Cataloging in Publication Data

Colgan, Michael,
    Protect Your Prostate

Includes index.
ISBN: 1-896817-25-4 (bound) - ISBN: 1-896817-17-3 (pbk.)

        1. **Prostate—Diseases—Alternative treatment. 2. Prostate--Diseases—Prevention. I. Title.**

RC899.C64 2000   616.6'5   C99-901625-3

Apple Publishing Company Ltd.
220 East 59th Avenue
Vancouver, British Columbia
Canada V5X 1X9   Tel (604) 214-6688   Fax (604) 214-3566

E-mail: books@applepublishing.com   Web Site: www.applepublishing.com

10   9   8   7   6   5   4   3   2   1

To Lesley my love

Abide with me

The best is yet to be

Also by Dr. Michael Colgan:

Electrodermal Responses
The Training Index
Your Personal Vitamin Profile
Prevent Cancer Now
Optimum Sports Nutrition
The New Nutrition: Medicine for the Millennium
Hormonal Health
Beat Arthritis

www.colganchronicles.com

Forewords

"For anyone who has had to navigate the largely uncharted areas of PSA numbers, Gleason scores, uncertain biopsies, and myriad and terrifying treatment options, Michael Colgan's approach in Protect Your Prostate *makes a very daunting challenge understandable and manageable — dare I say EASY!"*

Sir Michael Fay
CEO of Fay, Richwhite, who led New Zealand's
successful challenge for the America's Cup

"I first learned of Dr Michael Colgan while I was at the Salk Institute for Biological Studies in La Jolla, California. Dr Jonas Salk was so impressed with his early work, he personally wanted to sponsor Dr Colgan's research.

Later, when I served as Chairman of Psychology on the US Olympic Committee's Sports Medicine Council, I again was introduced to Michael Colgan's work as he helped prepare world class athletes for peak performance, both in nutrition and exercise physiology.

Fortunately, we became good friends. This has had a positive impact on my salmon and halibut fishing, but more critically, on my health and longevity.

As a conqueror of prostate cancer myself, I believe in and adhere to Dr Colgan's insights on prevention of prostate cancer and protection of the prostate, which should be learned by every male thirty years of age and older.

This book is a 'must read' for men who want quality and quantity of life, and who prefer to live by choice, rather than by chance."

Denis E Waitley, PhD
Renowned speaker and best-selling author
Author of The Psychology of Winning and
Empires of the Mind

v

Acknowledgments

My thanks to the many clients and friends who urged me to write this book, and to my staff who, with great patience and much merriment, held the whole thing together through all my fumblings and failings. I name the few who bore the brunt of the work, but extend my gratitude to all. Thanks to Marion Halliwell for her unfailing wit and laughter, and superb setting out and processing of the manuscript that make my scribbles look so good. Thanks to Cheryl Harrison and Eric Booth for editing the manuscript, and to Jocelyn Pettigrew, Steven Macramallah and my publisher Al Pazitch, for their patient support and incisive comment. And thanks most of all to my wife and fellow scientist, Lesley, my most trenchant critic and wisest advocate.

Introduction

A very famous man gave me the impetus to write this book, but I cannot name him because it would reveal that he has prostate disease. For more than a decade his prostate gave him increasing trouble, with a steadily rising score on the prostate specific antigen (PSA) test. But, like most of us, he refused the recommended surgery or even biopsy of the prostate, fearing it might worsen the problem.

In 1996 he began an individual nutrition program from the Colgan Institute. A year later, his PSA had dropped to almost normal and symptoms were negligible. His urologist, the best in his field, told me he had never seen such a reversal of prostate disease without complete removal of the prostate. He asked me exactly what we had done. In telling him, I realized that this brilliant physician was unaware of much of the research covered in this book. If someone as wise and educated as he was unaware, then many others might also benefit from these new discoveries in medical science.

Over the last 24 years, the Colgan Institute has developed the evolving nutritional program for prostate care documented herein. This program has helped to minimize the symptoms and progression of prostate disease in more than 1000 cases, and has enabled many more men to avoid it entirely. But remember, I am a scientist not a physician. So take this book and the medical references to your physician.

Physiology and biochemistry vary so much from one individual to the next, that only your physician, with detailed knowledge of your body, can decide whether the program is right for you. I hope it is, and wish you Godspeed in taming that prickly little gland.

Michael Colgan
Saltspring Island
August 1999

Contents

Forewords v

Acknowledgments vi

Introduction vii

1. Man-Made Plague 1

2. Case In Point 7

3. That Pesky PSA 11

4. The Changing Face Of Prostate Care...................15

5. Finasteride: A Real Advance 19

6. Cut The Calories 23

7. Cut The Fat 25

8. Eat Omega-3 Fats 29

9. Eat Carotenoids..33

10. Eat Lycopene 37

11. Take Vitamin C 41

12. Take Vitamin E 43

13. Take Selenium 47

14. Make And Take Vitamin D.................................51

15. Eat Soy 55

16. Saw Palmetto, Pygeum, Urtica...........................59

17. Eat Aged Garlic 65

18. Drink Green Tea 67

19. Zinc Your Prostate 71

20. A Daily Multi 75

21. How To Do It 77

References 83

About Dr Michael Colgan 95

Index 99

1

Man-Made Plague

In spring 1998, more than 7000 urologists from 72 countries gathered in Barcelona, Spain, for the largest urological convention ever. The main topics were erectile dysfunction and prostate disease.[1] The two are intimately connected, because half of all men who have prostate disease also have erectile dysfunction and other sexual problems.

By age 50, most men suffer some degree of prostate disease. They get **recurrent prostatitis** (inflammation of the prostate, usually caused by infection), or **benign prostatic hyperplasia** (BPH, overgrowth of the prostate gland), or both. By age 85, over 90% of men develop **prostate cancer**. Urologists are loathe to admit that earlier prostate disease eventually develops into cancer, because how it does so is still unclear. Nevertheless, the figures are undeniable.[1,2]

Until the last decade, degenerative conditions, such as prostate disease, were thought to be inevitable consequences of human aging. Recent discoveries, however, indicate they are much more the consequences of faulty nutrition and lifestyle. As this book will show you, *we* have created much of the prostate disease that now plagues our lives. The good news is: being man-made, the circumstances that create a lot of prostate disease are easy to discover — and to change. When they are changed by strong public health policies, a great deal of prostate disease will simply disappear. Until that occurs, which may take 30 years or more, you will have to take care of yourself.

Right now, virtually nothing is being done to prevent prostate disease. To the contrary, the increasing pollution of our environment, the destruction of nutrients in our food supply by mass agriculture and food processing, and the progressive adoption of unhealthy lifestyles continue to increase the degenerative burden on all tissues, including the prostate.

The incidence of prostate disease and the death rate from prostate cancer have soared in the last 20 years.[2] In America, during the present decade alone, the death rate for prostate cancer has grown to nearly twice that for breast cancer.[1] It is now the second leading cause of cancer death in American men, with about 335,000 new cases springing up every year.[2] With the right information, however, you should be able to prevent it for life.

The Structure Of Sexuality

Your prostate is a doughnut-shaped gland the size of a large walnut, lying just below your bladder. A small but vitally important tube, the **urethra**, descends from the bladder, passes through the doughnut hole of the prostate and continues through your penis. This tube carries your urine and also your sperm out of the body.

It's the prostate doughnut hole that causes most of the trouble. If it gets inflamed or squeezed because the prostate has grown too large, you get all sorts of waterworks problems — pain, irritation, increased urinary frequency, especially at night, and eventually urinary retention and kidney problems. These may be the least of your troubles, however, because prostate disease also whacks your sexuality.

Popular accounts describe the prostate simply as an accessory gland that secretes an alkaline fluid when you ejaculate, to protect the sperm from acidity of the urinary tract and of the female vagina. But it's a helluva lot more than that.

Figures 1 and 2 show the prostate in all its glory. Above the prostate lie two pouches, the **seminal vesicles,** which secrete a thick liquid full of fructose. This sugar provides energy for your sperm on their journey up the female reproductive tract. As you can see, the vesicles squirt out this liquid from ejaculatory glands deep inside the prostate, to mix with the thin, alkaline fluid that carries the sperm.

Also coming in from the top of the prostate are the two tubes of the **vas deferens** which run into the prostate doughnut hole after circling up and over it from the **epididymides** of the **testes**. Sperm manufactured in the testes flow to the epididymides to grow and mature there for a couple of weeks. From there they pass into the vas deferens tube which can store them for up to a month.

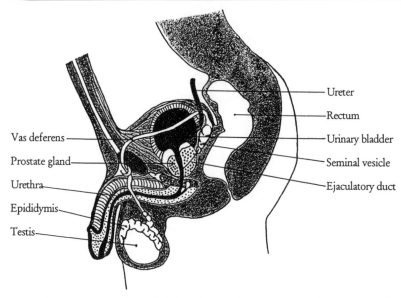

Figure 1. Sectional side view of prostate and associated structures.

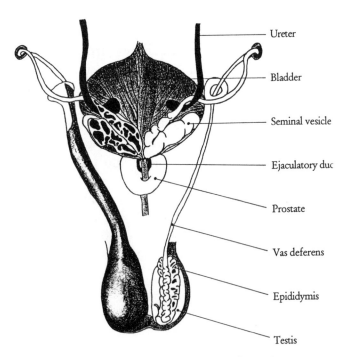

Figure 2. Prostate front view with surrounding tissue removed.

As you can see from Figures 1 and 2, ejaculation releases the sperm into the urethra deep inside the prostate. So the mixing and release of the whole shebang vital to male sexuality and human reproduction, all takes place in the doughnut hole of your prostate. No surprise then that prostate disease whacks your sexual potency hard — causing pain, impotence, loss of desire, and the inability to achieve orgasm — devastating all the vitality, well-being and confidence that are part of male virility.

You have a lot to lose if you let prostate disease get a grip, from loss of urinary function all the way to the myriad physical and mental aspects of healthy sexuality. Many men who have come to the Colgan Institute for help over the last 20 years didn't really mind having to get up five or six times a night to urinate, and could put up with the day-time symptoms as well. But very few could stand the loss of their virility. To keep yours, you need to know how to keep that prostate doughnut hole wide open and whistle clean.

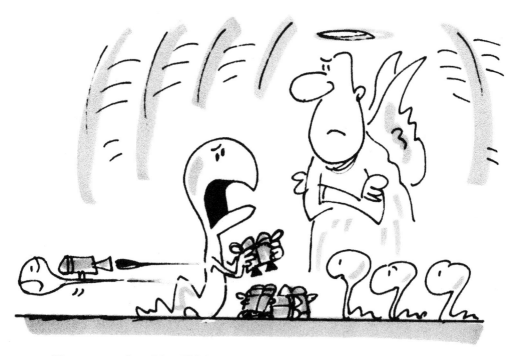

"It's no use you Complaints Division wallahs coming down here hassling me.
I'm having a devil of a job trying to get the kids through the prostate."

Case In Point

A recent case at the Colgan Institute illustrates the usual medical answer to the modern plague of prostate disease. Bob F— is a champion bodybuilder. He has great genetics and superb body symmetry. He always trains hard and gains muscle easily. But Bob never became a professional, because he trained for health as well as competition. He refused to take anabolic steroids and other bodybuilding drugs — the drugs that are necessary to gain that unnatural bulk of muscle that dominates the unhealthy sport of professional bodybuilding. Nevertheless, he became a regional champion, and proud of it.

In his late 30's, Bob noticed a mild but growing problem with his waterworks. He began to suspect BPH (benign prostatic hyperplasia). As we saw in Chapter 1, that's the medical gobble for overgrowth of the prostate gland. When it gets too big, the prostate chokes the hell out of your urinary stream and your sexuality.

Though BPH doesn't affect most men until after age 50, athletes tend to get it earlier in life. Unless they protect themselves, strength and bodybuilding athletes are affected most of all. Controlled epidemiological evidence is lacking, but a Colgan Institute analysis of athletes and of the research literature over the last 25 years indicates that male athletes in strength sports and track and field sports have at least an 80% chance of developing some degree of BPH by age 45. Why? Probably because athletes with high levels of muscle mass tend to have higher levels of testosterone than average. African Americans have some of the highest levels of testosterone and, predictably, suffer more BPH and more prostate disease than whites.[1]

On top of their genetic testosterone base, strength athletes also do everything they can with nutritional supplements and exercise to increase their testosterone even further. Part of that testosterone converts to **dihydrotestosterone** (DHT), the main culprit that causes your prostate to grow beyond normal size.

No wonder prostate cancer is common in users of anabolic steroids as they grow older.[2] These testosterone-derivative drugs load the body with dihydrotestosterone and cause the prostate to proliferate out of control. Even if you don't use drugs, if you are a strength athlete or even a weekend warrior, think hard before buying those purported anabolic supplements that litter muscle magazines. If they are at all effective, the ultimate reward for using them may be a slow and agonizing death.

Back to Bob. I'm telling you his case (with permission) because the same thing will likely visit you unless you take the right precautions. Bob was getting up four or five times a night to urinate. His urinary stream was dwindling. He felt urinary urgency numerous times a day but found it difficult to initiate urination. Then he began getting burning and irritation of the prostate after sex, then discomfort on ejaculation. Not a man who cared much for doctoring, he was finally forced by his symptoms to go for medical help.

The Shadow Of Cancer

After a thorough evaluation, his physician diagnosed BPH together with prostatitis, caused by a low-grade infection of the prostate. Prostatitis wasn't a bad guess, because over 90% of men get prostate infections some time or other. He put Bob on antibiotics and gave him a form to get a **prostate specific antigen (PSA) test**.

The antibiotics did nothing except make Bob nauseous, but the PSA was devastating. It came back at 9.4 ng/mL total PSA with free-PSA at 24%. The usual cut-off points for a clean bill of health are a PSA of 4.0 ng/mL with free-PSA above 25%. Diagnosis: a 65% chance of prostate cancer.

Bob couldn't believe it. How could this happen when he had spent his whole life in pursuit of health and strength? In deadly fear, he refused a confirming biopsy. His physician put him on androgen-blocking drugs to reduce his testosterone levels. He also strongly advised Bob to give up any supplements that might raise testosterone or stimulate output of steroid hormones from the pituitary or adrenals.

The list read like an advertising roster from a muscle magazine. It included ephedrine, yohimbe, HMB, DHEA, pregnenolone, androstenedione, glutamine, OKG, KIC, melatonin, acetyl-l-carnitine, and various herbals including ginseng, *ma huang*, hypericin and *tribulus terrestris*.

Worst of all, the physician advised Bob to give up heavy weight training because of its testosterone-raising effects. These were tough orders for a life-long natural bodybuilder to follow. But the PSA scores were so bad that Bob complied.

An Unnecessary Zombie

The androgen-blocking drugs drained his energy, his ability to maintain muscle and his sex drive. He cut workouts to a minimum. Over the next two years Bob lost 40 pounds of muscle, gained 26 pounds of fat, and became a physical and emotional wreck. His sex life declined to non-existent and his marriage went to hell. He was on three different anti-depressants and walked and talked like a zombie. But it did reduce his prostate problems.

At Bob's two-year examination, his physician detected a palpable lump on digital rectal examination of Bob's prostate, and insisted he have a multiple biopsy. Locked in major depression, Bob put it off again for months, fearful that if he did have localized prostate cancer, the biopsy would create needle tracks to leak it out. It's a legitimate fear. Relative to cancer cells, 'needle tracks' created by a biopsy are as big as a six-lane highway, along which cancer cells can migrate to other parts of the body.

Finally, when his PSA went over 11 ng/mL, Bob succumbed. The multiple biopsy came back *negative*. The lump was benign. The PSA and the physician's digit were not as accurate as commonly thought. Bob had spent three years in abject fear, had destroyed his love relationship and decimated the healthy, muscular body-of-a-lifetime — all for naught. That's when he came to me, with his physician's approval, to seek nutritional help. The first thing I explained to him was the dark side of the PSA.

3

That Pesky PSA

I was amazed that the four medical professionals Bob had seen all neglected to tell him that the PSA test has one of the highest false-positive rates of any medical test used today. It's bad business. In one well-controlled study, 78% of the men who scored between 4 ng/mL and 10 ng/mL on the PSA, *showed no trace of cancer when subjected to a biopsy.*[1] Imagine the effect on your life if you were one of those men falsely predicted by the PSA to be suffering from cancer.

Having read about the doubtful nature of the PSA in the popular press, Bob had expressed these fears to his physician. He was assured that the problem occurred only with the old PSA test. Bob was given the new version, which also compares the level of what is called **free-PSA** to **total PSA** in the blood. Free-PSA is lower in patients with prostate cancer. Bob's score was the wrong side of the cut-off line, indicating probable cancer.

But his physician was either unaware of the latest data on the free-PSA test, or else he didn't tell Bob about it. These data show that any power the new PSA test has to detect prostate cancer, disappears when prostate size exceeds 40 cubic centimeters.[2] Having both chronic prostatitis and BPH, Bob's prostate was BIG! But it was not cancerous.

Even If You Have A Tumor

Even if a localized prostate tumor is correctly detected by the PSA, it may not be a big problem. Autopsy studies of old men who die from other causes show that about *one man in every three* has a malignant tumor of the prostate — a tumor that was not involved in his death, was never treated, and probably did not cause any great health problem during his life.[3]

Prostate tumors are mostly slow growing and can sit there unnoticed and without symptoms for 20 to 30 years. That's probably the reason why there's no controlled evidence showing that PSA detection of cancer has had any effect whatsoever in reducing prostate disease, or in reducing deaths from prostate cancer.[4]

The evidence we do have points in exactly the opposite direction. The latest trial was published in the Journal of the American Medical Association in 1997, by prostate cancer expert Dr W Catalona and colleagues. They persuaded 322 healthy men, with *normal* results on the PSA, to undergo multiple prostate biopsies. (I don't know what they paid these heroes to irrevocably damage their prostates, but I wouldn't do it for a seven-figure sum.)

Of the 322 men, 73 (22%) were found to have prostate cancer.[5] The PSA test had failed utterly to detect even one of those cancers. Their PSA results had assured these men that they did not have prostate cancer. By failing to detect it, the PSA had falsely classified them as healthy. Consequently, they took no action to protect their prostates, allowing the disease to progress unchecked.

Worse, when you examine *correct* cancer diagnosis by the PSA, the rate of detection is also 22%![4] So, for every one hundred cases of real prostate cancer, the PSA detects only 22. And, from the study above, for each one of these 22 it also falsely detects a non-existent cancer in a healthy man. It's a crap shoot.

In sum, the PSA predicts as many non-existent cancers as it does real cancers, and misses most of the real cancers anyway. Despite all this hard evidence, The American Cancer Society (which positions itself as a medical authority, but is not) recommends the PSA, and has been largely responsible for the growth in use of this inaccurate and soul-destroying test. And some uninformed medicine men take it as gospel.

Don't Take Unnecessary Tests

I am pleased to see that the International Union Against Cancer advises *against* routine PSA testing.[6] So does the Canadian Task Force on Periodic Health Examinations.[7] The official health authority in the US, the Preventive Services Task Force, came down solidly against the PSA in its **Guide to Clinical Preventive Services**, and does *not* recommend its use.[3] If you doubt me, or if your physician is not fully aware of these official recommendations, you, he or she can access them on the internet at **http://158.72.20.10/pubs/guidecps/default.htm**.

Thumbs down on the PSA doesn't mean you can forget about your prostate. Latest figures show that prostate cancer is the second leading cause of cancer deaths of American men. Though we lack conclusive statistics, prostate cancer is probably the leading cause of cancer-related death in strength athletes, especially African Americans.[8] You definitely don't want BPH progressing into cancer.

Back to Bob for a final note. With the cooperation of his physician, I gave him a detailed program for restoration of his prostate and his manhood. It is almost identical to the program in this book. Now, nearly a year later, he has almost no symptoms, he's hitting the weights with gusto again, and smiling about his love-life. If you have the beginnings of a waterworks problem, or even the anticipation that you will develop one in the future, you need a similar program to protect yourself. Read on for all the details

4

The Changing Face Of Prostate Care

Most men do nothing to look after their prostates. They spend more time looking after their hair or teeth. Baldness or rotten choppers are seldom life-threatening, but a rotten prostate can kill you quick. As the second leading cause of cancer death in American men,[1] prostate cancer carries a lifetime risk nearly double that of breast cancer.[2] Whether you are 20 or 50, you should start taking care of that pesky little gland *today*.

Twenty years ago, the standard treatment for BPH and early stages of prostate disease was **transurethral resection of the prostate (TURP)**. In other words, whip it out. But the high rates of impotence, incontinence and other side-effects of this arcane little surgery, have prompted most urologists to seek other ways to remove chunks of overgrown prostate tissue.

Less invasive surgeries include transurethral incision (TUIP), electroevaporation, transurethral needle ablation, ultrasound destruction and laser prostatectomy. Surgeons today can even burn out bits of your prostate by microwaving. All these procedures are less effective than TURP and have almost as high rates of side-effects.[3] Whether or not you are still able to have erections on command, sex without pain, and urinate only when you want to, depends on the skill of the surgeon wielding the instruments. And prostate surgery is not reversible.

The Move To Drugs

In contrast, non-surgical drug therapies for BPH are both controllable and reversible. It is not surprising then that prostate medicine has moved in that direction. There are still many older physicians who were trained long ago to whip out the prostate at the first sign of trouble. If you run into one, get a second opinion. Chemo-control is a much better way to go.

Androgen-blockers, which eliminate bodily production of testosterone and dihydrotestosterone, cause rapid prostate shrinkage and rapid reduction of the prostate specific antigen (PSA) score. But they also cause almost 100% impotence. In addition, they carry a high rate of depression, because, as I have documented elsewhere, normal testosterone levels are essential for emotional well-being.[4] The only consolation is that the course of therapy is usually less than one year, and the side-effects are reversible.

Alpha-adrenoceptor antagonists, such as terazosin, alfuzosin, prazosin and tamsulosin, block testosterone and dihydrotestosterone receptor sites on prostate cells (and other body cells). They cause relaxation of the smooth muscle of the prostate, with consequent improved urination, ejaculation and reduction of symptoms of BPH. These drugs work quickly to relieve symptoms, but do nothing to reduce prostate size. Also, the symptom reduction is moderate, overall about 20%.[3]

Tamsulosin is the most promising of these drugs. The 1998 Urology Congress held in Barcelona, Spain, reviewed the latest data from large-scale trials involving 20,000 men. Unlike other alpha-blockers which affect a wide range of bodily functions, tamsulosin seems to be prostate-selective, so it has fewer side-effects. Nevertheless, symptom reduction remains moderate.[5]

The best drug news is the development of compounds that block an enzyme called **alpha-5-reductase,** thereby preventing testosterone from being converted to dihydrotestosterone. The leading drug is finasteride. We'll take a closer look at this clever man-made chemical in the next chapter.

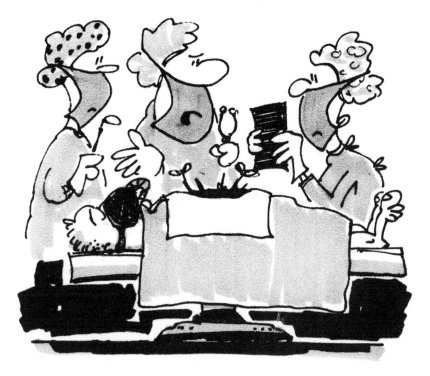

*"I know it says prostate resection Nurse Adams,
but he'll be a lot happier with an appendectomy."*

5

Finasteride: A Real Advance

Dihydrotestosterone is the main culprit in prostate overgrowth. The most effective drugs for prostate problems are those that block the enzyme **alpha-5-reductase**, which converts testosterone to dihydrotestosterone. The best and most extensively tested is **finasteride**. Finasteride works slowly, however, and needs to be taken for at least a year to achieve good results.[1] Over that period, it can reduce prostate size by up to 50%,[1,2] and cut the PSA score by half.[3]

In 1997, the Urology Department of Hospital University La Fe in Valencia, Spain, completed the longest trial to date of finasteride. From the seven-year study, researchers reported that symptoms improved by over 50% during the first year. They improved further (to 64%), while subjects continued on five milligrams per day of finasteride over the following six years. Prostate size was reduced overall by 26%. Some patients reported reduced libido and reduced sexual potency, but these side-effects occurred less frequently than with other drugs.[2]

The gold standard of experimental research, a double-blind, placebo controlled trial, has just confirmed this study, albeit with the more modest results that usually come from better controlled data. Headed by Dr M Marberger of the Department of Urology of the University of Vienna, Austria, multiple medical centers carried out this large study. It followed 3168 men with BPH over two years of finasteride treatment. Compared with placebo treatment, those given daily finasteride showed an average reduction in prostate size of 14% at one year and 15% at two years. The best news from these results is that men with the largest prostates benefited the most.[4] For men with BPH that is making their lives miserable, these studies are representative of the growing pile of data showing that a long-term course of finasteride provides relief.

Prescription Drug Problems

Despite its success, finasteride poses insurmountable problems for long-term use, problems that attend all man-made molecules. Finasteride did not exist on Earth during the evolution of the human species. Although it relieves BPH and even reverses prostate disease to a degree, we have no idea what else finasteride is doing to the body.

Over countless millennia, the evolving human body gradually developed the millions of mechanisms it uses today to deal with chemicals in its environment, mechanisms of such exquisite precision that science is still in the kindergarten of understanding them. But the body could develop these mechanisms only for chemicals that were present during evolution. It could not develop mechanisms to control the action of molecules that didn't exist during that time. It is therefore likely that man-made molecules, such as finasteride, will elude bodily controls and cause long-term detrimental side-effects. Unless you are desperate, think long and hard before putting them into your mouth.

If you conclude that its absence during evolution condemns *any* man-made molecule for long-term medical treatment, you are correct. Fortunately, thousands of informed physicians are now realizing that many, many of the prescription drugs being prescribed today are highly poisonous and should be used only as a last resort.[5]

Death By Prescription

The figures are irrefutable. On 15 April 1998, for example, the Journal of the American Medical Association reported on "adverse drug reactions" in American hospitals. Adverse drug reactions are not errors in medication. They are side-effects of drugs properly prescribed and used. In American hospitals alone, 2,216,000 patients suffered serious adverse drug reactions that killed 106,000 of them. That makes hospital prescription drugs the fourth leading cause of death in America today.[6] But don't worry. For the prostate there are potent alternatives to finasteride, which did exist during evolution, and which have no detrimental side-effects.

The second problem with finasteride and all the other prostate drugs, is that they do nothing to change the circumstances that produced the prostate disease in the first place. If you want to prevent it or reverse it, you better change those circumstances right away. Again, don't worry. Recent science has uncovered some of the main causes of prostate degeneration, and they are no more difficult to change than the way you do your hair.

> *"The first duty of the physician is to educate the masses **not** to take medicine."*
>
> Sir William Osler (1849-1919)
> Renowned British Physician

6

Cut The Calories

We eat too much. Despite all the low-fat, no-fat, God-forbid-there-ever-was-fat foods, all the low-cal meals, diet drinks, weight-loss schemes, chub clubs, and supposed fitness crazes, Western Society grows steadily fatter.

America is the worst. National Health Examination Surveys show that the average weight of Americans aged 18 – 74 has increased by about four pounds per decade since 1960.[1] Young adults are growing fattest of all. On 17 March 1994, the National Institutes of Health released figures showing that American men and women aged 25 – 30 had gained an average of 10 pounds over the previous eight years. With zero change in height or muscle, the increase is all flab.

What has this excess eating to do with prostate health? A lot! New research measuring total calorie intake shows a strong link between prostate cancer and the number of calories ingested daily, regardless of the type of food being eaten.

In a representative study, Dr S Andersson of the Department of Urology of Orebro Medical Center, Sweden, followed the diets of 526 newly diagnosed prostate cancer patients and 536 controls from 1989 through 1994. The highest quartile, that is the 25% of men with the highest calorie intake, increased their risk of prostate cancer by a whopping 70%.[2]   As is the case for numerous other diseases,[3] excess eating is a big health risk for prostate disease.

Step 1 to a healthy prostate: Cut the calories.

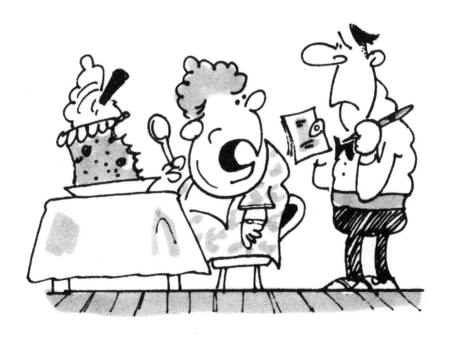

"I will have a latte but make sure it's with non-fat milk."

7

Cut The Fat

Mice and men are similar in numerous ways, one being their prostate glands. In the gobbledygook of physiologists: murine and human prostates are homologous in embryological origin and histological structure, and cancers in these tissues show similar characteristics. So the mouse is a reasonable model for investigating human prostate problems.

If you feed mice a typical Western diet, they develop prostate disease. In the latest study, researchers at Sloan-Kettering Cancer Center in New York, fed mice a typical Western human diet for 16 weeks. In that brief period, the mice developed overgrowth of cells in the prostate. Control mice, fed standard laboratory mouse chow, showed no prostate abnormalities. The crucial difference between these diets was the higher saturated fat content of the Western food.[1]

Human studies show similar findings. Dr A Whittemore and colleagues at Stanford University School of Medicine in California, examined the association of fat intake and prostate cancer in African-Americans (highest risk ethnic group), whites (high risk) and Asian-Americans (low risk), in Los Angeles, San

Francisco and Hawaii in the US, and Vancouver and Toronto in Canada. They compared 1600 patients with prostate cancer against 1600 healthy controls from 1987 to 1991. In all patient groups, prostate cancer was strongly correlated with saturated fat intake.

Also, about 25% of the difference in risk between the different ethnic groups was dependent on intake of saturated forms of fat. The African-Americans, who had the highest risk for prostate disease, ate the most saturated fat. The Asian-Americans, who had the lowest risk, ate the least saturated fat.[2]

Avoid Red Meats

The source of the fat is also important. A great deal of prostate disease is primarily an inflammatory condition. So anything that increases inflammation in body tissue should be avoided.

As I have documented elsewhere, meats, especially red meats, are not only high in saturated fats, but also contain high levels of **arachidonic acid**.[3] This preformed omega-6 fat is the precursor of a highly inflammatory compound in your body called **Prostaglandin E$_2$**. Men who eat large amounts of red meats are likely to create a pro-inflammatory condition in all their tissues, prostate included.

At the Colgan Institute, we have demonstrated the anti-inflammatory benefits of giving up red meat with many hundreds of athletes over the last 25 years. The levels of arachidonic acid in their bodies decline dramatically within weeks. Rates of connective tissue injury and other inflammatory conditions also decline by up to 70%.

Fat Breeds Fast Disease

Removing saturated fats from your diet is crucial, because they not only induce prostate disease but also speed its progression. The latest findings come from Dr I Bairati and team at Laval University in Quebec. They showed that prostate cancer grows more rapidly and aggressively in direct proportion to the amount of saturated fats in the patient's diet.[4] If you want a healthy prostate, get your fat intake below 25% of your calories, with saturated fats below 10%.

In this short account, I can't cite even a fraction of the other supporting studies now piled on my desk. But perhaps the summary statement of a leading prostate cancer specialist will convince you. Dr William Fair of the Sloan-Kettering Cancer Hospital in New York, said recently:

> We can take a man with a high PSA, put him on a diet containing only 15% fat calories and watch his PSA drop by 20% in three months.[5]

Remember, saturated fats are not only in meats and dairy products, but also include all hydrogenated vegetable fats in margarine, cooking oils and baked goods. I detail the problems of processed vegetable oils in my forthcoming book, **Essential Fats**.[6]

Step 2 to a healthy prostate: Cut the fat.

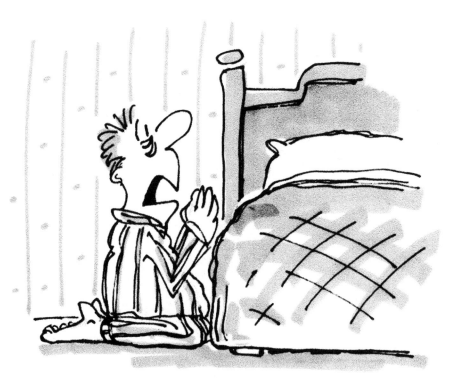

*"I swear I'll give up smoking, drinking, gluttony,
even my fat-back bacon if only you will let me pee."*

Eat Omega-3 Fats

The two essential fats are **linoleic acid** (omega-6) and **alpha-linolenic acid** (omega-3). These are the only two fats that your body cannot make but must obtain from your diet. They are essential for every cell membrane in the body, for the highly active structures of the brain, and numerous other organs and glands, including the prostate. Many folk are still unaware that the RDA Committee of the US National Academy of Sciences recommends a daily intake of 10 – 20 grams, a greater amount than for any essential vitamin or mineral.[1]

Most people do not get anywhere near this amount of intact essential fats. As documented in my forthcoming book, **Essential Fats**, modern processing of food oils damages what are called **double-bonds** in essential fats, the delicate bioactive chemical links that enable them to carry out their functions. Omega-3 fats have the most double-bonds and are the most easily damaged.[2]

In addition, because of their highly bioactive nature, oils containing high levels of omega-3 fats, such as flax or walnut, are more difficult to process on a mass scale. Because of this, large manufacturers have avoided them, thereby reducing the omega-3 content of the food chain. Numerous studies show that approximately 80% of Western diets have become deficient in intact omega-3 fats.[2]

Omega-6 Problems

Being somewhat more robust and more prevalent in the particular food oils popular today, omega-6 fats have survived the food oil industry better than omega-3s, thereby creating an unbalanced ratio of essential fats in Western diets. Although the overall intake of essential fats is too low, the vegetable fats we do get are primarily damaged omega-6s. In the absence of sufficient omega-3s, mounting evidence indicates that these omega-6 fats promote prostate disease.[3-6]

Numerous animal studies demonstrate pathological growth of the prostate when diets are high in processed linoleic acid (omega-6).[3,4] These findings are not really surprising, considering that modern processing changes the chemical structure of linoleic acid, so that it resembles that of saturated fat and becomes equally as damaging to the body.[2]

Recent studies in humans show similar effects,[4,5] especially when looking for evidence of prostate cancer rather than lesser forms of prostate disease. The most encouraging human and animal findings show that addition of omega-3 fats may afford protection against both the damaging effects of processed linoleic acid and prostate degeneration in general.[5,6]

The mechanisms of this protection are complex and beyond the scope of this short account. They involve both the contribution of omega-3 fats in building superior cell membrane structure in the prostate,[2] and in regulating the manufacture of other fats from omega-6, especially compounds called **eicosanoids**.[5] I document these mechanisms in more detail elsewhere.[2]

Overall, the evidence indicates that lifelong use of omega-3 fats is a wise strategy to protect your prostate. At the Colgan Institute, we use 20 grams (2 tbsp) of organic flax oil per day. At four parts omega-3 to one part omega-6, flax oil is the most potent commercial source of intact essential fats. Brands you can trust are **Barleans, Omega, Flora, Arrowhead Mills** and **Spectrum Naturals**.

A cautionary note – avoid cooking with oils that are high in heat-sensitive essential fats, such as flax oil. Similar to modern processing, high temperatures can transform them into *trans* fats, which are even more deadly than saturated fats.[2] Used as a salad dressing with vinegar, or for anything *uncooked*, flax oil is also quite palatable. I especially like the nutty taste of the Barleans brand, which makes a great base for gourmet salad dressings.

Step 3 to a healthy prostate: Use 20 grams of flax oil every day.

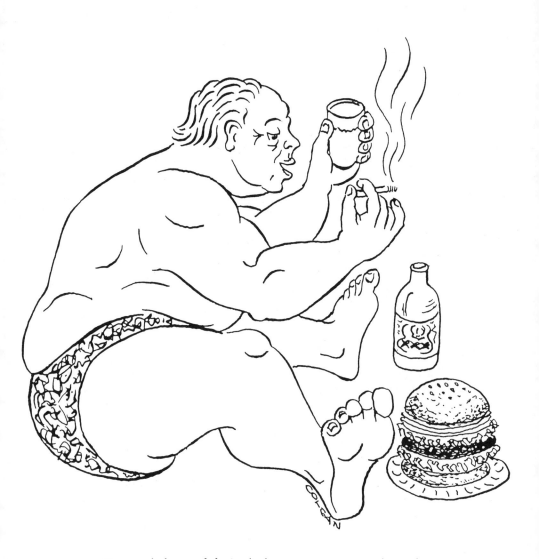

You need plenty of fat in the burgers to save your throat from the ciggies.

9

Eat Carotenoids

Researchers have long thought that **beta-carotene** and other precursors of vitamin A can protect the prostate, but they lacked definitive data to prove it. Muddying the water were several studies showing that the retinol form of vitamin A may *increase* prostate disease.[1]

The first clear evidence emerged in 1997 from the ongoing "Physicians Health Study," in which 22,000 male doctors are taking 50 milligrams (50,000 IU) of beta-carotene daily for 12 years. Control subjects (not given beta-carotene), who had low levels of beta-carotene in their blood at the start of the study, have increased their risk of prostate cancer by 33%.[2] In sharp contrast, physicians with low beta-carotene in their blood at the start of the study, who were in the group given beta-carotene, have *reduced* their risk of prostate cancer over the years by 36%.[2]

An heroic 30-year-long analysis of 1899 men with prostate cancer, completed in 1996 at Northwestern University Medical School in Chicago, offers further support. Survival over the whole 30 years was strongly linked with beta-carotene intake (and vitamin C intake) during that period.[3]

In 1997, British researchers showed how beta-carotene might perform this miracle. It increases the ability of the monocytes — foot soldiers of your immune system — to seek, identify and destroy cancer cells.[4]

These findings are especially important because of the low consumption of carotenoids in the diets of Americans, Canadians, Australians and New Zealanders. Despite frequent public recommendations from the US National Cancer Institute to eat five to nine servings of fruits and vegetables daily to prevent cancer, in 1995 Dr Susan Krebs-Smith of the Institute showed that less than one-third of Americans eat even four servings per day.[5]

As I documented in 1982, this situation has existed for many years[6] and is unlikely to change. It will probably worsen with the trend toward ever more processed foods, and the progressive destruction of food nutrients, including carotenoids.[7]

The Colgan Institute began using and recommending carotenoid supplements more than 25 years ago. We use supplements derived from natural beta-carotene because it has twice the biological activity of the synthetic form. Many folk on our programs, both men and women, have been using 50,000 IU per day for periods of 20 years or more, as a preventive strategy against the hormone-based cancers of the breast, endometrium, cervix and prostate.

We have seen no detrimental side-effects from these large supplements, not even yellowing of the skin, which some uninformed physicians warn against. The latest studies have just been reviewed by Professor John Hathcock, the pre-eminent world authority on nutrient toxicology. For normal folk, beta-carotene is completely non-toxic in these amounts.[8]

Step 4 to a healthy prostate: Take 25,000 IU of natural-source beta-carotene every day.

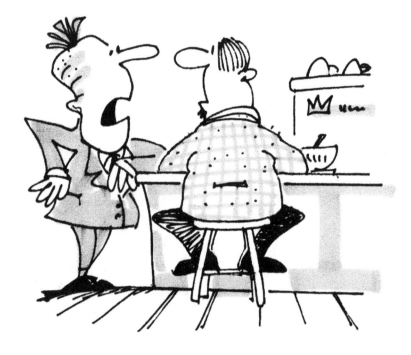

"I drink six glasses of carrot juice a day and it never turned my skin yellow."

Eat
Lycopene

Mediterranean countries have always had lower incidence of prostate and other hormone-based cancers than the rest of the West. Over the last two decades, studies have uncovered a direct link between this phenomenon and intake of tomatoes and tomato-based products.[1] The humble tomato has emerged in glory as a potent protector of the prostate.

Tomatoes get their color from a bright red carotenoid called **lycopene**. They are the main dietary source of this nutrient in Western society. Recent research shows clearly that lycopene protects prostate tissue.[2-6] Numerous test-tube and animal studies show that lycopene directly inhibits prostate tumor growth.[2]

Lycopene seems tailor-made for the job because, when eaten in sufficient quantities, it concentrates in the prostate (and testes and adrenals) at up to 20 times its concentration in other parts of the body. The level of lycopene in a well-supplied prostate falls nicely in the range that effectively suppresses tumor growth in cells in the laboratory.[3]

It also suppresses tumor growth in men. Human studies show that high intakes of tomato products and high serum levels of lycopene, dramatically reduce the risk of prostate disease.[4] One large study, recently published in the Journal of the National Cancer Institute, compared the lycopene intake of 48,000 men who were subjects in the "Health Professionals Follow-up Study" from 1986 to 1992. Men with the highest intakes of lycopene reduced their risk of prostate cancer by a massive 50%.[5,6]

Lycopene Harder To Get Than You Think

You may think you get plenty of lycopene from the abundance of tomato sauces, juices and dressings in our diets. Not so. A lot of that lycopene isn't bioavailable, because it is a highly lipid-soluble compound which is absorbed well only in the presence of fat.[1] Unless you eat some fat along with it, the lycopene may pass right through you.

Of course, you have to eat the right kind of fat. Mediterranean countries use liberal amounts of olive oil (a good oil) in their tomato products. The trend toward low-fat or no-fat foods, by using only the simple-minded and obsolete criterion of calorie content, has removed beneficial fats from Western diets, along with the bad fats. This chucking-the-baby-out-with-the-bathwater approach is bad news for your prostate.

Lycopene from raw tomatoes is not absorbed well either. Cooking releases the carotenoid, so cooked tomato products are the preferred source.[1] At the Colgan Institute, we mix a tablespoon of flax oil into pasta sauces or other tomato dishes, *after* they have been cooked, to aid in absorption of lycopene. In addition, we recommend supplementing your diet with 50 milligrams of pure lycopene every day.

Step 5 to a healthy prostate: Take 50 milligrams of lycopene every day and mix flax oil into tomato dishes after cooking.

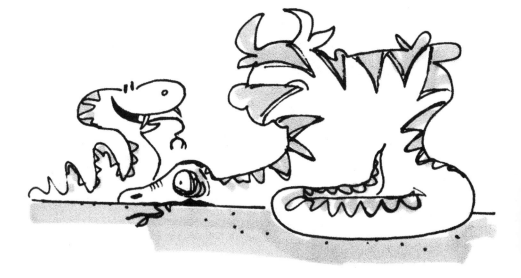

"Oh you must be the Full Monty Python."

11

Take Vitamin C

More than 100 controlled studies show strong effects of **vitamin C** in prevention and treatment of a variety of cancers, including hormone-based cancers of the breast, endometrium and prostate.[1-4] Studies of the killing action of vitamin C on prostate cancer cell lines have emphasized the antioxidant action of the nutrient, and have even shown how to enhance this action up to 20 times by the addition of vitamin K.[4,5]

Other studies, however, indicate that the potent effect of vitamin C involves multiple mechanisms in addition to its antioxidant action. These include: enhancing immune system action against cancer; neutralizing carcinogenic substances; and, destroying viruses and other infectious agents that promote cancer or speed its growth. Vitamin C also stimulates collagen formation to surround and encapsulate tumors to inhibit their progression.[1-4]

It is not surprising therefore, that a 30-year follow-up of prostate cancer, conducted by Dr M Daviglus and colleagues at Northwestern University Medical School in Chicago, found that overall survival was strongly linked to vitamin C intake (and beta-carotene intake).[6] Epidemiological studies also link vitamin C intake with prevention of prostate cancer.[2,3]

How Much Vitamin C?

The levels of vitamin C found effective in the above studies exceed by several orders of magnitude the amount that you can get from even an excellent diet. After reviewing all the data — including data on bioavailability, absorption and safety of vitamin C[3,7] — at the Colgan Institute, we use a daily intake of 2000 – 4000 milligrams of mixed mineral ascorbates, plus 500 milligrams of ascorbic acid.

As I document elsewhere, vitamin C works on the prostate only in conjunction with a full range of other essential nutrients.[3,7] Consequently, at the Colgan Institute, we use the vitamin C mix only in conjunction with a complete multiple vitamin/mineral formula, containing a wide range of other antioxidants, plus 50 micrograms of vitamin K_3. I debated this question on several occasions with Dr Linus Pauling during his life, the most brilliant biochemist of this century. It was not until he was in his late seventies that he agreed with me, and began seriously to add multiple vitamins and minerals to his own vitamin C regimen. Dare I say, had he done so earlier, we might still have the benefit of his continuing wisdom today.

Step 6 to a healthy prostate: As part of a multiple vitamin/mineral formula, take 1500 milligrams of mineral ascorbates, 500 milligrams of ascorbic acid, and 50 micrograms of vitamin K_3 every day.

Take Vitamin E

Research over the last three decades suggests that **vitamin E** affords protection against prostate cancer. Studies of cancer cell lines show clearly that vitamin E inhibits growth of a wide variety of cancers, an effect usually attributed to its general antioxidant action on the body. But recent evidence indicates that vitamin E acts more strongly against breast and prostate cancer cells than against other forms of cancer,[1] and that there is more than antioxidant action at work.[2]

In a series of recent studies, Dr K Israel and colleagues at the University of Texas in Austin showed that vitamin E even inhibits growth of strong, aggressive lines of prostate cancer cells which cause metastasis (spread of the cancer to other organs) in humans. When it combines with these cells, vitamin E stimulates secretion of a growth-inhibiting chemical called **transforming growth factor-beta**.[2] This chemical is a normal mechanism used by your body to prevent growth of pathological cells. That it can be prodded into action against cancer, even aggressive metastatic cancer, by a non-toxic essential nutrient is good news indeed.

Despite such encouraging findings, until now vitamin E has received mixed reviews from cancer experts, because of a lack of definitive data on human cases. This situation changed in 1996 with the publication of a 17-year follow-up of the "Basel Prospective Study." The study measured plasma levels of vitamin E and other nutrients in 2,974 men in Basel, Switzerland. Results verified earlier work, showing that there are fewer deaths from prostate cancer among men with high levels of vitamin E in their blood.[3]

Then in 1998, results of the "Alpha-tocopherol, Beta-carotene Cancer Prevention Study" were published in various journals. This trial gave 29,000 male smokers either 50 milligrams of vitamin E, 20 milligrams of beta-carotene, both, or a placebo for eight years. Results showed that those receiving vitamin E developed one-third fewer prostate cancers than the placebo group. Vitamin E also reduced prostate cancer mortality by 41%.[4,5] With this strong evidence, vitamin E supplementation is a wise addition to preventive maintenance of the prostate.

Vitamin E For Prostatitis

Even if you do not have prostate cancer or BPH, vitamin E can be very helpful. Prostatitis affects 90% of men at some time in their lives. One big cause of prostatitis is **lipid peroxidation** — oxidative damage, mainly to cell membranes, caused by free radicals. Recent research from Russia indicates that, because of its strong antioxidant action in lipids, vitamin E supplementation is an effective addition to treatment of chronic prostatitis.[5]

If you do decide on vitamin E supplementation, don't use any old vitamin E. In the past, many of the studies and human cases have been compromised by supplements containing synthetic dl-alpha-tocopherol, which is cheaper than the natural-source d-alpha-tocopherol. Though both are designated on labels as equivalent doses of vitamin E in milligrams (mg) or International Units (IU), the synthetic dl form is a mix of eight different **isomers** of vitamin E, only one of which is as bioactive as the natural-source d-alpha-tocopherol. Numerous studies now show that natural-source vitamin E is up to five times more absorbable, active and easily retained in the body.[6-8]

At the Colgan Institute, we use up to 800 IU of **d-alpha-tocopherol succinate**, because this is the most stable form of the natural-source vitamin E, and is the form found to be most effective against prostate cancer cells.[2,9]

Step 7 to a healthy prostate: As part of a multiple vitamin/mineral formula, take up to 800 IU of d-alpha-tocopherol succinate every day.

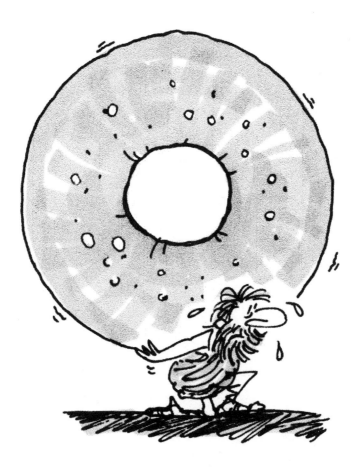

13

Take
Selenium

In 1982, I reported that **selenium** is scarce in the soils of 10 American states plus the district of Columbia.[1] It is similarly scarce in the soils of large areas of Australia and most of New Zealand, to the extent that livestock have to be supplemented with the mineral to attain normal health.[2] For humans, however, selenium has been largely ignored. It was not included in the table of Recommended Dietary Allowances (RDA) until 1989,[3] 35 years behind the evidence of its importance to our health.

Your body cannot make selenium. You must obtain this essential mineral from your diet. If the soils are deficient, then the produce and livestock raised on those soils are deficient also. And so are you.

Average adult selenium intake in America is 108 micrograms per day, which means that about one-quarter of the adult population gets less than 50 micrograms per day.[4] The very conservative

Recommended Dietary Allowance for selenium is 70 micrograms for men, and 55 – 65 micrograms for women. So even in terms of the RDA, selenium deficiency is widespread.

Though studies are sparse, the data that we do have on nutrition status in specific diseases, and in the elderly, frequently show selenium intakes of less than the RDA.[5] This problem is compounded when you consider that the amount of selenium found effective in long-term prevention and treatment of various diseases is 200 – 600 micrograms per day.

Very few folk get those amounts, and scientists have suspected for many years that selenium deficiency may be a major cause of the progression of prostate disease. Blood selenium levels are much lower in patients whose prostate disease has progressed into cancer, than in patients who have BPH but no cancer.[6]

Selenium Kills Prostate Cancer Cells

Selenium also dramatically inhibits the growth of prostate cancer cells. In a recent representative study, Dr C Redman and colleagues at the University of Arizona in Tucson showed that selenium, in the form **selenomethionine**, prevented growth of both prostate and breast cancer cell lines in a dose-dependent manner. The most important finding from this study is that it didn't take a lot. Selenomethionine inhibited cancer cell growth at levels of 45 – 130 microM. Such levels are easily achieved in the blood with supplementary oral selenomethionine in a completely non-toxic dose. To damage normal cells takes about one thousand times this dose.[7]

This evidence is crucial, because it confirms earlier work that shows prostate cancer cells are much more sensitive to destruction by selenium than are normal cells. So selenium may be able to kill prostate cancer with no toxicity and no side-effects, exactly the sort of "magic bullet" against cancer that researchers are always seeking.

New controlled trials of selenium in human subjects confirm these findings. Dr G Combs and colleagues at Cornell University in Ithaca, New York, gave 1300 patients either 200 micrograms of selenium per day or a placebo, from 1983 to 1990, then followed them until 1993. The group receiving selenium developed much less prostate cancer and had a much lower incidence of, and mortality from, all forms of cancer.[8]

The latest study is a large, randomized, double-blind trial carried out by Dr L Clark and team of the University of Arizona, Tucson, on a sample from the Combs study above. Of the 843 subjects who had normal PSA levels (less than 4 ng/mL) at the start of the study, the control group, who were not given selenium, developed prostate cancer at *four times* the rate of the selenium group.[9]

In this short account, I have space to give you only these few examples of the evidence that selenium is a potent inhibitor of prostate disease. I have tried to present the latest studies that are representative of the trend of evidence of more than 50 studies over the last 20 years. I hope it is sufficient to convince you.

The most potent form of selenium is the organically bound **selenomethionine,** produced by the **Nutrition 21** company in San Diego, California. For all men over 40 on our programs, especially for men who are experiencing any symptoms of prostate degeneration, the Colgan Institute uses a daily supplement of 200 – 600 micrograms.

Step 8 to a healthy prostate: As part of a multiple vitamin/mineral formula, take 200 micrograms of selenomethionine every day.

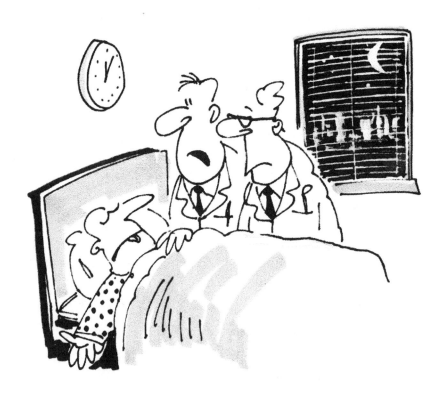

*"That's the trouble with magic bullets against cancer,
___at midnight they turn back to pumpkins."*

14

Make And Take Vitamin D

Every day we are bombarded with pseudo-medical advice to avoid all direct exposure of your skin to sunlight, especially from makers of cosmetics. This advice has little to do with health, and is just one more example of the distortion of science to serve commercial greed. Numerous studies do show that *excessive* exposure to sunlight damages the skin by causing silent and unfelt oxidation in the dermis (the underlying, living layer of skin) resulting in aging of the skin and increased risk of skin cancer. No controlled evidence exists, however, showing that similar damage occurs with moderate sun exposure.

Nevertheless, commercial misinformation has persuaded many people to stay out of the sun. This is not a good idea, because without moderate sun exposure (20 – 30 minutes per day, depending on latitude) your body cannot form the essential seco-steroid hormone, still popularly known as **vitamin D**. A great deal of recent evidence shows that vitamin D is a potent protector against breast and prostate cancer.[1]

Because pharmaceutical companies cannot patent natural molecules such as vitamin D — so cannot secure the commercial protection necessary to ensure their profit margin — most of the research on vitamin D and prostate cancer uses man-made derivatives of vitamin D, which can be patented. Nevertheless, of the natural forms of vitamin D studied, research shows that **vitamin D$_3$**, also called **calcitriol** or **cholecalciferol,** is as potent as most of the derivatives and can prevent prostate cancer in animals.[1,2]

In one of the latest studies, Dr R Getzenberg and team at the University of Pittsburgh Cancer Institute in Pennsylvania, infected rats with deadly metastatic prostate cancer cells. Half the rats were then given vitamin D$_3$. In the group supplemented with the vitamin, the cancer grew much slower and they developed fewer metastases.[2]

Begin Vitamin D Early

Vitamin D$_3$ also strongly inhibits growth of some human prostate cancer cells. These cancer cells are categorized by their degree of transformation from normal cells, which means roughly by how deadly they have become. The **LNCaP** line is the least deadly, the **PC-3** line is more deadly, and the **DU-145** line is the mostly deadly of the commonly studied prostate cancer cells. Vitamin D_3 easily stops growth in the LNCaP cells,[3] and moderately inhibits growth in PC-3 cells.[4]

The most transformed and most deadly cell line, DU-145, is almost completely resistant to vitamin D. New evidence indicates the DU-145 can bypass vitamin D because it has become **androgen-independent**. That is, it has transformed to become independent of hormones, and no longer needs testosterone or dihydrotestosterone to support its growth. The less transformed and less deadly cell lines are still androgen-dependent.[5]

This important information indicates that you should start using vitamin D_3 before prostate cancer begins, and certainly before it progresses into an aggressive metastatic form. Once you develop androgen-independent cancer in the prostate, it's a much more difficult job to stop it.

The latest study in humans illustrates the benefits of early use of vitamin D. Dr C Gross and team at Stanford University School of Medicine in California, studied patients with early prostate cancer that had recurred following radiation or surgical treatment. The recurrence was signaled by rising PSA levels. To minimize side-effects on body calcium and parathyroid hormone levels, they gave the patients a small initial daily dose of 0.5 micrograms of vitamin D_3 and slowly increased the dose to 2.5 micrograms. Over the six to 15 months of vitamin D_3 use, results showed a significant reduction of PSA activity.[6]

Vitamin D_3 has one drawback. In the range of 1.5 – 2.5 micrograms daily it can cause the body to lose calcium.[6] So, as with all nutritional strategies suggested herein, you should use it only under the guidance of your physician, who can monitor your bloodwork on a regular basis. At the Colgan Institute, we use 2.5 – 5.0 micrograms of vitamin D_3 per day as a preventive measure. We have done so now for more than 20 years, with very few cases of calcium loss. Nevertheless, individuals differ in their biochemistry so much that our program should not be adopted by anyone without the approval of, and regular monitoring by, their physician.

We also advocate daily exposure of the body to the sun for 20 – 30 minutes so that vitamin D can form on your skin and be absorbed for use by all your organs. Even if the sky is overcast, you still get the benefit.

Step 9 to a healthy prostate: As part of a multiple vitamin/mineral formula, take 100 IU of vitamin D_3 and expose your body to 20 minutes of sunlight every day.

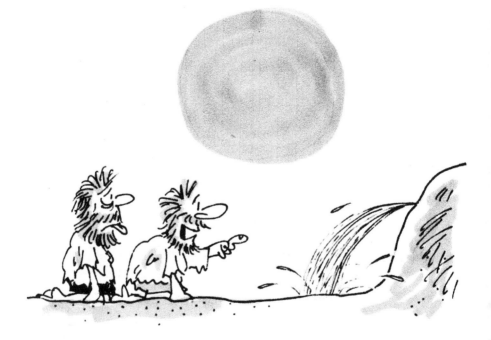

"Things are lookin up. We're loaded with vitamin D and there's the water."

15

Eat Soy

Breast and prostate disease are much less prevalent in the Orient than in America, Britain, Canada, Australia and New Zealand.[1,2] Death from prostate cancer in Japan is a very rare event. For many years, researchers have suspected that the high intake of traditional soy products by Oriental people somehow protects them. But the beneficial substances in soy that do the trick were not pinpointed until the late 1980s.

Most promising from current research is a soy flavonoid, an isoflavone called **genistein**, first isolated in 1987.[3] Also protective are other soy isoflavones, including **diadzein** and **equol,** and a sterol that occurs in numerous plant foods called **beta-sitosterol.**[4]

In test-tube studies, genistein inhibits the growth of some prostate cancers very well. More important, it also prevents BPH. Even if you do not have prostate problems, eating foods with a high genistein content as an habitual part of your diet, may stop the whole progressive cycle of prostate disease before it starts.

Begin Using Soy Early

More evidence for starting to use soy products before cancer strikes comes from studies on rats. In one recent representative study, from the University of Notre Dame in Indiana, rats were fed a soy-based diet containing high amounts of the isoflavones genistein and diadzein. Control rats were fed a low-isoflavone diet. Both groups were then deliberately infected with a potent prostate carcinogen.

The rats fed isoflavones developed fewer cancers and remained disease-free much longer than the control rats.[5] But feeding the same isoflavones to rats *after* the cancer was established, dramatically reduced the benefits. So it's likely that a soy diet works much better for prevention of prostate disease than for a cure.

Sources Of Genistein

The concentration of genistein (and its derivative genistin) varies widely in different soy foods. Traditionally prepared Japanese fermented soybean products, **tofu** (bean curd), **miso** (bean paste) and **natto** (fermented soybeans) contain high levels, ranging from 100 – 950 micrograms of genistein per gram of food. Soy isolate powders, especially the **Supro** brand made by Protein Technologies International in St Louis, Missouri, also contain up to 950 micrograms per gram. In contrast, "Westernized" soy foods, such as fake soy bacon or hamburger, may contain less than 20 micrograms of genistein per gram.[6]

Oriental populations consume eight to 80 milligrams of genistein per person per day, whereas Western populations consume only one to three milligrams.[3,6] In order to get the health benefits, you should use only the most potent sources of genistein, and make them a regular part of your diet.

At the Colgan Institute, we use traditional Japanese soy foods plus a whey/soy protein drink containing Supro soy isolate powder.

Step 10 to a healthy prostate: Drink a high isoflavone soy protein shake every day and eat Oriental soy foods.

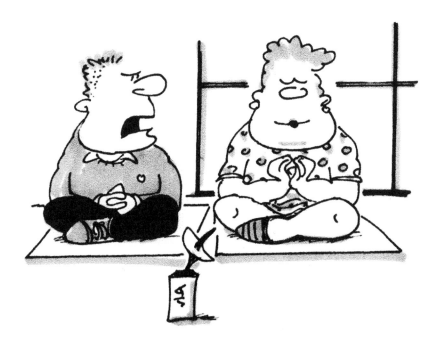

"I don't mind eating the tofu Martha, but this has gone too far."

16

Saw-Palmetto, Pygeum, Urtica

In Chapter 5 we looked at the problems with the drug finasteride and I promised you an equally effective alternative for reducing BPH that has virtually no side-effects. It consists of three plants: **saw palmetto**, **pygeum** and plain old **stinging nettle**. Various combinations of these herbals are medically approved in Europe, and have been widely prescribed for two decades as effective treatment of BPH.

In America, however, pharmaceutical companies exert heavy pressure on physicians and medical schools in the form of grants, endowments and endless promotions, to persuade them to recommend patented, highly profitable, man-made drugs. The effects of financial and career incentives trickle down to the plethora of non-peer-reviewed medical school newsletters, medical magazines, television and radio programs, and popular media articles, many of which are financially supported by pharmaceutical interests. The general thrust of these public communications is to praise prescription drugs and vilify non-patentable herbals as useless, dangerous, or at least "unproven."

Television news services are especially gullible to the professionally produced, pre-canned film provided free by the drug-makers. These pieces save TV news people much time and money. They are often aired verbatim, without critical comment, especially if they come from one or another of the organizations calling themselves "medical news services." These services pose as independent scientific clearing houses, when in reality they are owned and operated by pharmaceutical interests. Consequently, the public continues to be misled. Having no pharmaceutical profits to pursue, and accepting no grants or other incentives from drug companies, the Colgan Institute is free to report the science as it is documented in the peer-reviewed medical literature.

Saw Palmetto

Saw palmetto extract comes from two varieties of fan palm, *Sabal serrulata* and *Serenoa repens,* that grow wild across the southern United States and in parts of Europe. So this prostate remedy is inexpensive to produce and widely available. And it works!

In the '60s, European scientists established that saw palmetto extract reduces levels of dihydrotestosterone in the prostate (the leading culprit in BPH), mainly by inhibiting the enzyme 5-alpha-reductase.[1,2] This is exactly what finasteride does too.

Since then, more than 20 controlled studies, five of them in the last decade, have shown that saw palmetto can do a lot more, including inhibiting detrimental effects of estrogen and progesterone on the prostate, and deactivating inflammatory compounds. With these additional attributes, saw palmetto can reduce prostate size, reduce inflammation, relieve prostatitis, improve sexuality and lessen other symptoms of prostate disease.[3-7]

One recent study compared saw palmetto directly with finasteride. Both treatments were equally effective in reducing the conversion of testosterone to dihydrotestosterone. The saw palmetto, however, had fewer side-effects.[5] For long-term safety, and certainly for economy, saw palmetto is the better bet.

Pygeum

Pygeum (*Pygeum africanum*) is the powdered bark of a common African evergreen tree. It offers benefits similar to saw palmetto, but works by different biochemical mechanisms. It's major active ingredient is the sterol **beta-sitosterol** (also found in soy). Beta-sitosterol has only weak effects on sex hormones, but it helps to lower high cholesterol, which some researchers believe is implicated in prostate disease.

In a recent double-blind study, representative of the growing evidence, 200 men with troublesome BPH were given either 60 milligrams per day of beta-sitosterol or a placebo, for three months. Those receiving the herbal showed improved urine flow and relief of other symptoms.[8] Various companies are now producing supplements of purified beta-sitosterol from a variety of plant sources for the treatment of prostate problems. Until solid studies support a particular preparation, however, I would stick with pygeum.

Two other recent studies report the important finding that pygeum not only relieves symptoms of BPH, but can also reduce the size of the prostate.[9,10] Overall, this research offers reasonable evidence that pygeum may not only relieve prostate symptoms, but also help to *reverse* the course of prostate disease. It is a worthy addition to your armamentarium.

Urtica

Nettle (*Urtica dioica*) grows wild just about everywhere. The evidence for nettle extract is not as strong as for the other two herbs, but it is still substantial. The first controlled double-blind trial of merit was done in 1985. It showed significant relief of symptoms of BPH.[11]

In current trials, nettle is usually combined with saw palmetto or pygeum. The latest study compared one of these combinations directly with finasteride. In a large multi-center, double-blind, clinical trial, Drs J Sokeland and J Albrecht of the University of Munster in Germany studied 543 men with BPH. They gave the men either 320 milligrams of saw palmetto extract plus 240 milligrams of nettle extract, or the recommended dose of finasteride, for one year. The two treatments were equally effective in relieving symptoms. The herbals, however, had virtually none of the side-effects of impotence, reduced sexual function and headache that are common with finasteride.[12] The choice is yours, but I know which choice is mine.

At the Colgan Institute, we have used these three herbals for more than a decade, in both treatment and prevention of prostate disease. Either alone or in combination, we use a lipophilic extract of saw palmetto, standardized for 90% fatty acids, at doses of 300 – 1000 milligrams per day. We use a lipophilic extract of pygeum bark, standardized for 13% total sterols, at doses of 100 – 300 milligrams per day. And we use a lipophilic extract of stinging nettle in doses of 250 – 750 milligrams per day. Excellent products conforming to these standards are sold by the **Life Extension Foundation** based in Florida.

Step 11 to a healthy prostate: Take extracts of saw palmetto 600 milligrams, pygeum 200 milligrams and nettle 500 milligrams every day, half in the morning and half in the evening.

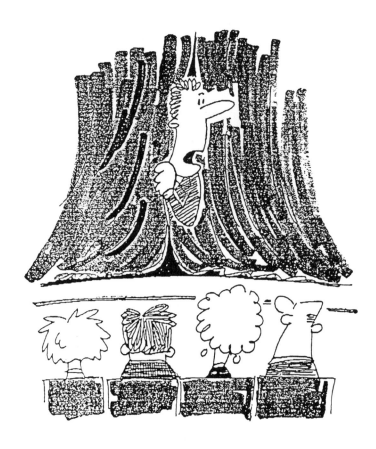

Is there a naturopath in the house?

17

Eat Aged Garlic

Organically grown garlic that is aged for at least one year in the traditional Oriental way, dramatically increases its content of a sulfur compound called **S-allylmercaptocysteine**. Some sulfur compounds in garlic, especially those in fresh garlic, are unstable, and others are too rapidly inactivated in the human body to be of value for the prostate. S-allylmercaptocysteine is both stable and biologically active for a considerable amount of time.[1]

In 1997, Drs Richard Rivlin and John Pinto, researchers at the Sloan-Kettering Cancer Center in New York, showed that S-allylmercaptocysteine rapidly breaks down testosterone in prostate cancer cells, and does so by a chemical route that does not produce dihydrotestosterone. This action slowed the growth of the cancer cells in culture by as much as 70%. It also reduced production of PSA, which is itself a promoter of prostate cancer growth.[1-3]

These important findings have just been confirmed by Dr G Sigounas and team at East Carolina University School of Medicine in Greenville, North Carolina. They report that S-allylmercaptocysteine reduces growth of human prostate cancer cells (and breast cancer cells). This non-toxic herbal kills many of these cancer cells, yet has little effect on normal human cells.[4]

It works by inhibiting an enzyme called **ornithine decarboxylase**, which is required for the cancer cells to produce proteins.[3] This discovery of specific cancer-killing action by an inexpensive food is an enormous boon in prostate care. And, with a tip o' me hat to Fry and Laurie, we are ever on the lookout for enormous boons.

Unfortunately, you cannot achieve the same effect using raw garlic, cooked fresh garlic, or pills made from fresh garlic. Their content of S-allylmercaptocysteine is insignificant. Nevertheless, the amount of the crucial compound used in the study above suggests that you can achieve the same blood levels by using garlic that has been hung in the traditional manner, or by taking aged garlic pills, as a regular part of a prostate maintenance program.

At the Colgan Institute, we use up to 4.0 grams of **Kyolic** aged garlic extract per day, and have done so for more than a decade without side-effects. We use the Kyolic supplement made by the **Wakunaga** company of Mission Viejo in California. Not only do they age their garlic in the traditional manner for a year, but they also add S-allyl-cysteine during the aging process, which gets converted to S-allylmercaptocysteine. And it doesn't leave a garlic smell on your breath.

Step 12 to a healthy prostate: Take 1.0 gram aged garlic extract every day.

18

Drink Green Tea

You have an enzyme in your body called ornithine decarboxylase. In the presence of testosterone and its derivatives, this sneaky little beggar is a potent stimulus for formation of proteins that make up your cells. For years, researchers have wondered whether ornithine decarboxylase might overstimulate the prostate, causing it to run amok. These suspicions have just been confirmed. In June 1999, Dr R Mohan and colleagues at Case Western Reserve University in Cleveland, Ohio, showed conclusively that prostate cancers, and fluid from overgrown prostates, contain abnormally high levels of ornithine decarboxylase.[1]

Compounds that inhibit ornithine decarboxylase should therefore reduce the growth of testosterone-dependent prostate cancer cells. One such is the S-allylmercaptocysteine from garlic, discussed in Chapter 17. Green tea also contains potent inhibitors of ornithine decarboxylase. These compounds, called **polyphenols**, effectively stop growth of various types of cancer in animal experiments.[2]

Further new research at Case Western Reserve University, has just shown that green tea polyphenols inhibit growth of testosterone-dependent prostate cancer in the test tube, in rats and in mice.[3] Human trials are on the way.

Stopping DU-145

Green tea does a lot more than inhibit one sneaky little cell-growth enzyme. One of the polyphenols it contains has multiple protective actions against BPH and prostate cancer. In medical gobble, this non-toxic herbal compound is called **epigallocatechin-3-gallate**. It inhibits the enzyme 5-alpha-reductase, which converts testosterone to the more dangerous dihydrotestosterone.[4] You will recall that the prescription drug finasteride, covered in Chapter 5, makes its claim to fame by doing the same.

Unlike the drug, the green tea polyphenol has additional actions that are good news to anyone with serious prostate cancer. As I discussed in Chapter 14, the most deadly prostate cancer is the DU-145 cell line. DU-145 is prostate cancer which has become androgen-independent. That is, it continues its deadly growth even if all testosterone and its derivatives are removed from the prostate. If you have cells similar to DU-145 in your prostate, conventional hormone-blocking medicines are useless. Recent work at the Mayo Clinic in Rochester, Minnesota, and elsewhere, shows that epigallocatechin-3-gallate kills DU-145 very nicely.[5,6] Again, human trials are on the way.

In The Real World

Don't let these complex laboratory experiments confuse you. Green tea has a lot of real world support as well. Two good epidemiological studies indicate that men who regularly drink green tea have a lower risk of prostate cancer.[2,6]

China is a very large nation of diverse peoples, most of whom live at what we call subsistence level. They eat diverse foods, but one unifying factor is the nation-wide use of green tea as a regular part of the daily diet. As you might expect, with many poor people and little to spend on advanced medicine, they have a poor health record for many diseases. But the incidence of prostate cancer in China is the lowest in the world.[7] Coincidence? I do not think so.

Step 13 to a healthy prostate: Drink green tea as a regular part of your daily diet.

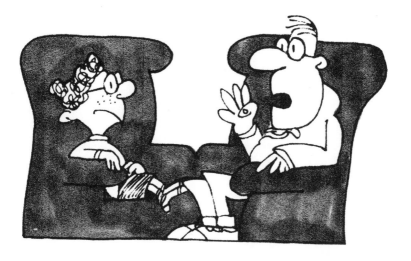

"Men have four problems in life son. Women, money, booze, and prostate."

19

Zinc Your Prostate

Many more nutrients are involved in prostate health than those covered in preceding chapters. I have covered only those nutrients which have prostate-specific benefits when taken in larger amounts than can be obtained from your food. The final one of these is the essential mineral **zinc**. You need plenty of zinc. In the healthy prostate, zinc is concentrated at much higher levels than in other parts of your body.[1] This extreme level has multiple protective functions in the prostate and reproductive system.

One important function is to prevent prostate infection. In 1976, Dr W Fair was the first to show that zinc has strong antibacterial action in the prostate.[2] He showed also that prostatic zinc levels of men with chronic prostatitis averaged only 50 mug/ml, compared with 448 mug/ml in healthy men. Further, the decline in prostate zinc is not *caused* by infection, but *precedes* it.[2] Once an infection is established, zinc supplements alone do not shift it, because they do not restore prostate zinc levels.[2] All nutrients work in synergy, so taking zinc alone will not work.

Killing off the bacteria with antibiotics is also of little use, except as temporary symptomatic relief. Immediately after you stop taking the drugs, bacteria re-enter the prostate to start a new infection cycle. Antibiotics are somewhat like United Nations peacekeeping forces. Once they are withdrawn, the nationals go to war again.

The best strategy is to maintain a permanent peacekeeping force by taking adequate zinc every day as a part of a complete vitamin/mineral supplement. If you are unlucky enough to develop prostatitis, then you may need antibiotic reinforcements for a while to get it under control. But it's the zinc home guard that's going to keep you healthy afterwards.

An additional strategy to reduce bacterial infection is to empty the prostate of seminal fluid at least once a week by sexual intercourse or, if necessary, by masturbation. Studies indicate that prostate fluid may become stagnant and provide a breeding ground for any of the 200 bacteria known to cause prostatitis.[3]

Zinc And Prostate Cancer

Zinc does not prevent BPH, because men with this level of prostate disease have even higher prostate zinc levels than healthy men.[4] Two lines of evidence suggest that the rise in zinc with BPH may represent a bodily defense mechanism to prevent the disease from progressing into prostate cancer. First, in test-tube studies, zinc kills prostate cancer cells when used at equivalent levels to those found in normal prostates and in BPH.[5] Second, in prostate cells, zinc uniquely prevents oxidation of a compound called **citrate**, which is produced in high levels by the prostate for a variety of purposes. High levels of citrate oxidation enable prostate cancer cells to grow rapidly.[1,6,7]

Prostate cancer may well represent a failure of zinc protection, because prostate zinc levels in men with this form of cancer are very low — about 10% of normal.[8] Even though zinc levels in the prostate are mostly under hormonal controls, one likely cause of low prostate zinc is insufficient zinc in your diet over an extended period of time.

In the US, insufficient dietary zinc is widespread. The average zinc intake of the American diet is below the RDA of 15 milligrams, even if you eat as much as 3000 calories per day.[9] Detailed studies of actual zinc intake reveal a daily intake of only 8.6 milligrams.[10] That's one big invitation to prostate disease.

At the Colgan Institute, we use 20 – 50 milligrams per day of zinc picolinate, the form of zinc most easily absorbed. This amount may be criticized as possibly interfering with copper metabolism. Some 39,000 people have taken programs with us in the past 25 years, and we have not seen a single case of such interference. The crucial factor that prevents such a problem occurring is: we never advise taking zinc alone. Like all other vitamins and minerals, zinc should be used only as part of a complete supplement of essential nutrients.

Step 14 to a healthy prostate: As part of a multiple vitamin/mineral formula, take 20 milligrams of zinc picolinate every day.

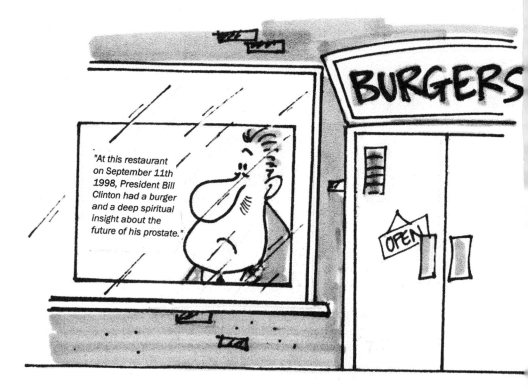

20

A Daily Multi

On 8 April 1998, the Food and Nutrition Board of the US Institute of Medicine, which sets the Recommended Dietary Allowances (RDAs) as an affiliate of the US National Academy of Sciences, made the most important public announcement of its 58-year history. After half a century of steadfast denial, it finally admitted that Americans do not get sufficient vitamins and minerals from their food supply, and recommended that almost all Americans should eat a good diet, *and take daily vitamin/mineral supplements.*[1]

The Colgan Institute has presented strong evidence supporting such a recommendation since 1974. We have taken many brickbats for our stance. It's nice to be vindicated. There is no longer any doubt that you should take a complete vitamin/mineral complex every day to protect against multiple deficiencies caused by the low levels of these micronutrients in our food.

Make sure the formula is complete, because the essential nutrients work properly only in synergy with each other. As I document in my book **Optimum Sports Nutrition,** if even one is missing or deficient, then it compromises the action of all the others.[2] The Colgan Institute has designed and recommends the multi-vitamin/mineral formulas found in the **Colgan Institute** AM/PM Paks.

Step 15 to a healthy prostate: Take a complete multiple vitamin/mineral complex every day.

21

How To Do It

It goes without saying that protection of your prostate is part of the necessary preventive maintenance of your whole body. Without maintenance, your body will inevitably break down into premature degeneration and disease. I cover the best strategies for general maintenance in other books.[1-3] Here it suffices to say that you should follow the latest medical recommendations for health.

Avoid foods and other lifestyle items that irritate and damage your organs. Don't smoke, and stay away from smokers. Don't drink more than a glass or two of wine a day. Especially be careful of cheap wine and liqueurs because they are full of damaging chemicals. Don't eat highly spiced foods or hot curries. Avoid salted foods, red meats, preserved meats, all high-fat foods and processed vegetable oils, except for essential fats.[2] Avoid highly processed carbohydrates.[4] Drink plenty of pure water, preferably distilled. Eat moderately.

Follow the National Cancer Institute recommendation to eat five to nine servings of fruit and vegetables per day to prevent cancer.[5-7] Base your diet on organically grown fruits and vegetables, nuts, seeds and whole grains, using meats and fish as garnish rather than vegetables, nuts, seeds and whole grains, using meats and fish as garnish rather than the main part of the meal. Get your veggies, nuts, seeds and grains fresh, because their content of nutrients disappears rapidly with storage and processing.[3,8]

Stay lean for life because bodyfat is the harbinger of many diseases, including prostate disease.[3] And get some regular weight-bearing exercise. We now know for certain that weight-bearing exercise prevents many cancers, including breast and prostate cancer.[3,9]

Program Summary

If you don't have any prostate problems, or only the beginnings of them, the lifestyle and supplements noted herein may seem a bit troublesome and expensive. If they do, then contact your local chapter of the Prostate Society and ask a few folk who have real prostate disease. They will tell you that relief from it is worth all the gold of Midas.

With the approval and cooperation of their physicians, at the Colgan Institute, we have applied various combinations of our nutritional program to over 1000 men suffering from prostate disease. We have seen some outstanding results and virtually no side-effects. Before you adopt anything described herein, however, take this book and the medical references to your physician. You can obtain copies of the abstracts of all the studies listed in the References section from medical libraries by using Internet Grateful Med, Medline at http://igm.nlm.nih.gov. It costs you only the internet connection time.

You must consult your physician because *this book is a compilation of the latest science, it is not a treatment.*

Individuals vary so much in their biochemistry and physiology, that only your physician, with intimate knowledge of your body, can decide if this program is right for you. I hope it is, because the time to begin to protect your prostate is — *now.*

I wish you Godspeed in taming that pesky little gland. To aid you on your way, the 15 steps to protect your prostate are summarized in Table 1 on the next page. The full Colgan Institute Prostate Supplement Program is summarized in Table 2 on the page following.

Table 1: 15 Steps to a Healthy Prostate

Step 1	Cut the calories.
Step 2	Cut the fat.
Step 3	Use 20 grams of flax oil every day.
Step 4	Take 25,000 IU of natural-source beta-carotene every day.
Step 5	Take 50 milligrams of lycopene every day and mix flax oil into tomato dishes *after* cooking.
Step 6	Take vitamin C (1500 milligrams of mineral ascorbates and 500 milligrams of ascorbic acid) and 50 micrograms of vitamin K$_3$ every day.*
Step 7	Take up to 800 IU of d-alpha-tocopherol succinate, vitamin E, every day.*
Step 8	Take 200 micrograms of selenomethionine every day.*
Step 9	Take 100 IU of vitamin D$_3$ and expose your body to 20 minutes of sunlight every day.*
Step 10	Drink a high isoflavone soy protein shake every day and eat Oriental soy foods.
Step 11	Take extracts of saw palmetto 600 milligrams, pygeum 200 milligrams and nettle 500 milligrams every day, half in the morning and half in the evening.
Step 12	Take 1.0 gram aged garlic extract every day.
Step 13	Drink green tea as a regular part of your daily diet.
Step 14	Take 20 milligrams of zinc picolinate every day.*
Step 15	Take a complete multiple vitamin/mineral complex every day.

---

* These nutrients should be included in your multi-vitamin/mineral complex. If they are not, or if they are included in lesser amounts, supplements may be taken to meet the daily dosages recommended here.

Table 2: Colgan Institute Prostate Supplement Program

Morning shake (made in blender)

- 8 ounces non-fat milk
- 30 grams ion-exchange whey protein concentrate plus high-isoflavone soy protein
- 2 tablespoons organic flax oil
- Fresh fruit to taste

Take with shake

- Multi-vitamin/mineral morning pack
- 25,000 IU beta-carotene
- 50 milligrams lycopene
- extracts of saw palmetto 300 milligrams, pygeum 100 milligrams and nettle 250 milligrams
- 500 milligrams of aged garlic extract

Noon At least two cups of green tea with lunch.

Evening

- Two cups of green tea with dinner
- Multi-vitamin/mineral evening pack
- extracts of saw palmetto 300 milligrams, pygeum 100 milligrams and nettle 250 milligrams
- 500 milligrams of aged garlic extract

Please note - Your morning and evening multi-vitamin/mineral packs combined should include **at least** the following amounts of nutrients:
- 1500 milligrams mineral ascorbates, vitamin C
- 500 milligrams ascorbic acid, vitamin C
- 50 micrograms vitamin K_3
- Up to 800 IU d-alpha-tocopherol succinate, vitamin E
- 200 micrograms selenomethionine
- 20 milligrams of zinc picolinate
- 100 IU vitamin D_3

© The Colgan Institute, San Diego, CA, 1998

References

Chapter One: Man-Made Plague

1. Philips P. Reports at European Urology Conference reflects issues of interest to aging men. **JAMA**, 1998;279:1333-1335.
2. Brawley OW. Prostate carcinoma incidence and patient mortality: the effects of screening and early detection. **Cancer**, 1997;80:1857-1863.

Chapter Two: Case In Point

1. Brawley OW. Prostate carcinoma incidence and patient mortality: the effects of screening and early detection. **Cancer**, 1997;80:1857-1863.
2. Colgan M. **Optimum Sports Nutrition**. New York: Advanced Research Press, 1993.

Chapter Three: That Pesky PSA

1. Catalona WJ, et al. Measurement of prostate specific antigen in serum as a screening test for prostate cancer. **New Engl J Med**, 1991;324:1156-1161.
2. Meyer A, et al. Factors influencing the ratio of free to total prostate-specific antigen in serum. **Int J Cancer**, 1997;74:630-636.
3. Report of the US Preventive Services Task Force. **Guide To Clinical Preventive Services, 2nd Ed**. Alexandra, VA: International Medical Publishing, 1996.
4. Stern S, et al. Detection of prostate and colon cancer. **JAMA**, 1998;280:117-118.
5. Catalona WJ, et al. Prostate cancer detection in men with serum PSA concentrations of 2.6-4.0 ng/mL and benign prostate examinations.

Enhancement of specificity with free PSA measurements. **JAMA,** 1997;277:1452-1455.

6. Miller AB. Screening for cancer: state of the art and prospects for the future. **World J Surg,** 1989;13:79-83.
7. Canadian Task Force on the Periodic Health Examination, 1991, Update 3: secondary prevention of prostate cancer. **Can Med Assoc J,** 1991;145:413-428.
8. Ventura SJ, et al. Births and deaths: United States, 1996. **Mon Vital Stat Rep,** 1997:46(Suppl 2):1-40.

Chapter Four : The Changing Face Of Prostate Care

1. Stern S, et al. Detection of prostate and colon cancer. A decision analytic view. **JAMA,** 1998;280:117-118.
2. Krahn MD, et al. Screenings for prostate cancer. **JAMA,** 1994;272:773-780.
3. Tammela T. Benign prostate hyperplasia. Practical treatment guidelines. **Drugs Aging,** 1997;10:349-366.
4. Colgan M. **Hormonal Health.** Vancouver: Apple Publishing, 1996.
5. Philips P. Reports at European Urology Conference reflects issues of interest to aging men. **JAMA,** 1998;279:1333-1335.

Chapter Five : Finasteride: A Real Advance

1. Lieber MM. Pharmacologic therapy for prostatism. **Mayo Clinic Proc,** 1998;73:590-596.
2. Martinez Sarmiento M, et al. Treatment of benign prostatic hyperplasia with finasteride. Results after 7 years of follow-up. **Actas Urol Esp,** 1997;21:105-110.
3. Pannek J, et al. Influence of finasteride on free and total serum prostate specific antigen levels in men with benign prostate hyperplasia. **J Urol,** 1998;159:449-453.
4. Marberger MJ. Long-term effects of finasteride in patients with benign prostate hyperplasia: a double-blind, placebo-controlled multi-center study. **Urology,** 1998;51:677-686.

5. Moore TJ, et al. Time to act on drug safety. **JAMA**, 1998;279:1571-1573.
6. Lazarou J, et al. Incidence of adverse drug reactions in hospitalized patients: a meta-analysis of prospective studies. **JAMA**, 1998;279:1200-1205.

Chapter Six : Cut The Calories

1. Wurtman RJ, (ed). **Human Obesity**. New York: New York Academy of Sciences, 1987.
2. Andersson SO, et al. Energy, nutrient intake and prostate cancer risk: a population-based, case-control study in Sweden. **Int J Cancer**, 1996;68:716-722.
3. Colgan M. **The New Nutrition: Medicine For The Millennium.** Vancouver: Apple Publishing, 1995.

Chapter Seven : Cut The Fat

1. Xue L, et al. Induced hyperproliferation in epithelial cells of mouse prostate by a Western-style diet. **Carcinogenesis**, 1997;18:995-999.
2. Whittemore AS, et al. Prostate cancer in relation to diet, physical activity and body size in blacks, whites and Asians in the United States and Canada. **J Natl Cancer Inst**, 1995;87:652-661.
3. Colgan M. **Beat Arthritis**. Vancouver: Apple Publishing, in press.
4. Bairati I, et al. Dietary fat and advanced prostate cancer. **J Urol**, 1998;159:1271-1275.
5. American Prostate Society, **Update**, Summer/Fall 1997:1.
6. Colgan M. **Essential Fats**. Vancouver: Apple Publishing, in press.

Chapter Eight : Eat Omega-3 Fats

1. Food and Nutrition Board, National Academy of Sciences. **Recommended Dietary Allowances**. Washington DC: National Academy Press, 1989.
2. Colgan M. **Essential Fats**. Vancouver: Apple Publishing, in press.

3. Willett WC. Specific fatty acids and risks of breast and prostate cancer: dietary intake. **Am J Clin Nutr**, 1997;66:1557S-1563S.
4. Godley PA, et al. Biomarkers of essential fatty acid consumption and risk of prostatic carcinoma. **Cancer Epidemiol Biomarkers Prev**, 1996;5:889-895.
5. Rose DP. Dietary fatty acids and cancer. **Am J Clin Nutr**, 1997;66:998S-1003S.
6. Rose DP. Dietary fatty acids and prevention of hormone-responsive cancer. **Proc Soc Exp Med**, 1997;216:224-233.

Chapter Nine : Eat Carotenoids

1. Giovannucci E, et al. Intake of carotenoids and retinol in relation to risk of prostate cancer. **J Nat Cancer Inst**, 1995;87:1767-1776.
2. Stampler M. Paper Presented at the Annual Meeting of the American Society of Clinical Oncologists, Denver,CO, 19 May 1997.
3. Daviglus ML, et al. Dietary beta-carotene, vitamin C, and risk of prostate cancer: results from the Western Electric Study. **Epidemiology**, 1996;7:472-477.
4. Hughes DA , et al. The effect of beta-carotene supplementation on the immune function of blood monocytes from healthy male non-smokers. **J Lab Clin Med**, 1997;129:309-317.
5. Krebs-Smith S. US adults' fruits and vegetables intakes 1989 to 1991: a revised baseline for the Healthy People 2000 objective. **Am J Pub Health**, 1995;85:1623-1629.
6. Colgan M. **Your Personal Vitamin Profile**. New York: William Morrow and Company, Inc., 1982.
7. Colgan M. **The New Nutrition: Medicine For The Millennium.** Vancouver: Apple Publishing, 1994.
8. Hathcock JN. Vitamins and minerals, efficacy and safety. **Am J Clin Nutr**, 1997;66:427-437.

Chapter Ten: Eat Lycopene

1. Weisburger JH. Evaluation of the evidence on the role of tomato products in disease prevention. **Proc Soc Biol Med**, 1998;218:140-143.

2. Stahl W, Sies H. Lycopene: a biologically important carotenoid for humans? **Arch Biochem Biophys**, 1996;336:1-9.
3. Clinton SK, et al. Cis-trans lycopene isomers, carotenoids and retinol in the human prostate. **Cancer Epidemiol Biomarkers Prev**, 1996;5:823-833.
4. Gerster H. The potential role of lycopene for human health. **J Am Coll Nutr**, 1997;16:109-126.
5. Giovannucci E, et al. Intake of carotenoids and retinol in relation to risk of prostate cancer. **J Nat Cancer Inst**, 1995;87:1767-1776.
6. Stampler M. Paper Presented at the Annual Meeting of the American Society of Clinical Oncologists, Denver, CO, 19 May 1997.

Chapter Eleven: Take Vitamin C

1. Colgan M. **Hormonal Health**. Vancouver: Apple Publishing, 1996.
2. Head KA. Ascorbic acid in the prevention and treatment of cancer. **Altern Med Rev**, 1998;3:174-186.
3. Colgan M. **The New Nutrition: Medicine for the Millennium**. Vancouver: Apple Publishing, 1994.
4. Maramag C, et al. Effect of vitamin C on prostate cancer cells in vitro; effects on cell number, viability and DNA synthesis. **Prostate**, 1997;32:188-195.
5. Venugopal M, et al. Synergistic anti-tumour activity of vitamins C and K3 against human prostate carcinoma cell lines. **Cell Biol Int**, 1996;20:787-797.
6. Daviglus ML, et al. Dietary beta-carotene, vitamin C, and risk of prostate cancer: results from the Western Electric Study. **Epidemiology**, 1996;7:472-477.
7. Colgan M. **Optimum Sports Nutrition**. New York: Advanced Research Press, 1993.

Chapter Twelve: Take Vitamin E

1. Sigounas G, et al. dl-alpha-tocopherol induces apoptosis in erythroleukemia, prostate and breast cancer cells. **Nutr Cancer**, 1997;28:30-35.

2. Israel K, et al. RRR-alpha-tocopheryl succinate inhibits the proliferation of human prostatic tumor cells with defective cell cycle/differentiation pathways. **Nutr Cancer**, 1995;24:161-169.
3. Eichholzer M, et al. Prediction of male cancer mortality by plasma levels of interacting vitamins: 17-year follow-up of the Prospective Basel Study. **Int J Cancer**, 1996;66:145-150.
4. Heinonen OP, et al. Prostate cancer and supplementation with alpha-tocopherol and beta-carotene: incidence and mortality in a controlled trial. **J Nat Cancer Inst**, 1998;90:440-446.
5. Tarasov NI, et al. Correction of abnormal lipid peroxidation in treatment of chronic prostatitis. **Urol Nefrol (Mosk)**, 1998;Jan/Feb:38-40.
6. Ingold KU, et al. Biokinetics of and discrimination between dietary RRR- and SRR-alpha-tocopherols in the male rat. **Lipids**, 1987;22:163-172.
7. Traber MG, et al. RRR- and SRR-alpha-tocopherols are secreted without discrimination in human chylomicrons, but RRR-alpha-tocopherol is preferentially secreted in low-density-lipoproteins. **J Lipid Res**, 1990;31:675-685.
8. Acuff RV, et al. Relative bioavailability of RRR- and all rac-alpha-tocopheryl acetate in humans: studies using deuterated compounds. **Am J Clin Nutr**, 1994;60:397-402.
9. Pryor WA. **Vitamin E and Carotenoid Abstracts, 1996**. Lagrange, 1L:Veris, 1997.

Chapter Thirteen: Take Selenium

1. Colgan M. Soils low in selenium. **Science**, 1981;214:744
2. Mertz W, (ed). **Trace Elements in Humans and Animal Nutrition 5th Edition**. New York: Academic Press, 1986.
3. Food and Nutrition Board of the National Academy of Sciences. **Recommended Dietary Allowances**. Washington DC: National Academy Press, 1989.
4. Pennington JA, et al. Selected minerals in food surveys. **J Am Diet Assoc**, 1984;84:771-780.
5. Schmuck A, et al. Analyzed dietary intakes, plasma concentrations of zinc, copper, and selenium, and related antioxidant enzyme activities in hospitalized elderly women. **J Am Coll Nutr**, 1996;15:462-468.

6. Hardell L, et al. Levels of selenium in plasma and glutathione peroxidase in erythrocytes in patients with prostate cancer and benign hyperplasia. **Eur J Cancer Prev**, 1995;4:91-95.
7. Redman C, et al. Inhibitory effect of selenomethionine on the growth of three selected human tumor cell lines. **Cancer Lett**, 1998,125;103-110.
8. Combs GF Jr., et al. Reduction of cancer risk with an oral supplement of selenium. **Biomed Environ Sci**, 1997;10:227-234.
9. Clark LC, et al. Decreased incidence of prostate cancer with selenium supplementation: results of a double-blind cancer prevention trial. **Brit J Urol**, 1998;81:730-734.

Chapter Fourteen: Make And Take Vitamin D

1. Studzinski GP, Moore DC. Sunlight — can it prevent as well as cause cancer? **Cancer Res**, 1995; 55:4014-4022.
2. Getzenberg RH, et al. Vitamin D inhibition of prostate adenocarcinoma growth and metastasis in the Dunning rat prostate model system. **Urology**, 1997;50:999-1006.
3. Fife RS, et al. Effects of vitamin D_3 on proliferation of cancer cells in vitro. **Cancer Lett**, 1997;120:65-69.
4. Wang X, et al. The in vitro effect of vitamin D_3 analogue EB-1089 on a human prostate cancer cell line (PC-3). **Brit J Urol**, 1997;80:260-262.
5. Zhao Xy. 1 alpha, 25-dihydroxyvitamin D_3 actions in LNCaP human prostate cancer cells are androgen-dependent. **Endocrinology**, 1997;138:3290-3298.
6. Gross C, et al. Treatment of early recurrent prostate cancer with 1,25-dihydroxyvitamin D_3 (calcitriol). **J Urol**, 1998;159:2035-2040.

Chapter Fifteen: Eat Soy

1. Geller J, et al. Genistein inhibits the growth of human-patient BPH and prostate cancer in histoculture. **Prostate**, 1998;34:75-79.
2. Morton MS, et al. Measurement and metabolism of isoflavonoids and lignans in the human male. **Cancer Lett**, 1997;114:145-151.

3. Barnes S, et al. Rationale for the use of genistein-containing soy matrices in chemoprevention trials for breast and prostate cancer. **J Cell Biochem Suppl**,1995;22:181-187.
4. Kennedy AR. The evidence for soybean products as cancer preventive agents. **J Nutr**, 1995;125:733S-743S.
5. Pollard M, Luckert PH. Influence of isoflavones in soy protein isolates on development of induced prostate-related cancers in L-W rats. **Nutr Cancer**, 1997;28:41-45.
6. Fukutake M, et al. Quantification of genistein and genistin in soybeans and soybean products. **Food Chem Toxicol**, 1996;34:457-461.

Chapter Sixteen: Saw Palmetto, Pygeum, Urtica

1. Duker EM, et al. **Planta Med**, 1989;55:587.
2. Champault G, et al. Medical treatment of prostatic adenoma. Controlled trial: PA 109 vs placebo in 110 patients. **Ann Urol**, 1984;6:407-410.
3. Braeckman J, et al. The extract of Serenoa repens and benign prostatic hyperplasia: A multi-center open study. **Curr Ther Res**, 1994;55:776-785.
4. Dathe G, et al. Phytotherapy of benign prostatic hyperplasia (BPH) with extractum Serenoa repens. **Urologie B**, 1991;31:220-223.
5. Strauch G, et al. Comparisons of finasteride and Serenoa repens in the inhibition of 5-alpha-reductase in healthy male volunteers. **Eur Urol**, 1994;26:247-252.
6. Bracher F. Phytotherapy of benign prostatic hyperplasia. **Urologe A**, 1997;36:10-17.
7. Gerber GS. Saw palmetto (Serenoa repens) in men with lower urinary tract symptoms: effects on urodynamic parameters and voiding symptoms. **Urology**, 1998;51:1003-1007.
8. Berges R. Randomized placebo-controlled, double-blind clinical trial of beta-sitosterol in patients with benign prostatic hyperplasia. **Lancet**, 1995;345:1529-1532.
9. Mathe G, et al. A Pygeum africanum extract with so-called phyto-estrogenic action markedly reduces the volume of true and large prostatic hypertrophy. **Biomed Pharmacother**, 1995;49:341-343.

10. Carani C, et al. Urological and sexual evaluation of benign prostatic disease using Pygeum africanum at high doses. **Arch Ital Urol Nefrol Androl**, 1991;63:341-345.

11. Vontobel HP, et al. Results of a double-blind study on the effectiveness of ERU (extractum radicis urticae) capsules in conservative treatment of benign prostatic hyperplasia. **Urologe A**, 1985;24:49-51.

12. Sokeland J, Albrecht J. Combination of Sabal and Urtica extract vs finasteride in benign prostatic hyperplasia (Aiken stages I-II) Comparison of therapeutic effectiveness in a one-year double-blind study. **Urologe A**, 1997;36:327-333.

Chapter Seventeen: Eat Aged Garlic

1. Raloff J. Aged garlic could slow prostate cancer. **Science News**, 1997;151:1.

2. Rivlin R, Pinto JT. Paper presented at the Annual Meeting of the Society for Experimental Biology, New Orleans, April 1997.

3. Pinto JT, et al. Effects of garlic thioallyl derivatives on growth, glutathione concentration and polyamine formation of human prostate carcinoma cells in culture. **Am J Clin Nutr**, 1997;66:398-405.

4. Sigounas G, et al. S-allylmercaptocysteine inhibits cell proliferation and reduces the viability of erythroleukemia, breast and prostate cancer cell lines. **Nutr Cancer**, 1997;27:186-191.

Chapter Eighteen: Drink Green Tea

1. Mohan RR, et al. **Clin Cancer Res**, 1999;5:143-147.

2. Myers CE. Differentiating agents and non-toxic therapies. **Urol Clin North Am**, 1999;26:341-351.

3. Gupta S, et al. Prostate cancer chemoprevention by green tea: in vitro and in vivo inhibition of testosterone-mediated induction of ornithine decarboxylase. **Cancer Res**, 1999;59:2115-2120.

4. Liao S, Hiipakka RA. Selective inhibition of steroid 5-alpha-reductase by tea epicatechin-3-gallate and epigallocatechin-3-gallate. **Biochem Biophys Res Comm**, 1995;214:833-838.

5. Paschka AG, et al. Induction of apoptosis in prostate cancer cell lines by the green tea component epigallocatechin-3-gallate. **Cancer Lett**, 1998;130:1-7.
6. Ahmad N, et al. Green tea constituent epigallocatechin-3-gallate and induction of apoptosis and cell cycle arrest in human cells carcinoma cells. **J Natl Cancer Inst**, 1997;89:1881-1886.
7. Gupta S, et al. Prostate cancer chemoprevention by green tea. **Semin Urol Oncol**, 1999;17:70-76.

Chapter Nineteen: Zinc Your Prostate

1. Costello LC, Franklin RB. Novel role of zinc in the regulation of prostate citrate metabolism and its implications in prostate cancer. **Prostate**, 1998;35:285-296.
2. Fair WR, et al. Prostatic antibacterial factor. Identity and significance. **Urology**, 1976;7:169-177.
3. Hennenfont B. Prostatitis. **American Prostate Quarterly,** 1995;3:9.
4. Dutkiewicz S. Zinc and magnesium serum levels in patients with benign prostatic hyperplasia (BPH) before and after prazosin therapy. **Mater Med Pol**, 1995;27:15-17.
5. Iguchi K, et al. Induction of necrosis by zinc in prostate carcinoma cells and identification of proteins increased in association with this induction. **Eur J Biochem**, 1998;253:766-770.
6. Costello LC, et al. Zinc inhibition of mitochondrial aconitase and its importance in citrate metabolism of prostate epithelial cells. **J Biol Chem**, 1997;272:28875-28881.
7. Liu Y, et al. Prolactin and testosterone regulation of mitochondrial zinc in prostate epithelial cells. **Prostate**, 1997;30:26-32.
8. Zaichick VYe, et al. Zinc in the human prostate gland: normal, hyperplastic and cancerous. **Int Urol Nephrol**, 1997;29:565-574.
9. Hambridge KM, et al. Zinc. In: Mertz W. ed. **Trace Elements in Human and Animal Nutrition 5th Edition Vol 2.** New York: Academic Press, 1986:1-137.
10. Holden JM, et al. Zinc and copper in self-selected diets. **J Am Diet Assoc**, 1979;75:23-28.

Chapter Twenty: A Daily Multi

1. **Washington Post**, 8 April 1998.
2. Colgan M. **Optimum Sports Nutrition**. New York: Advanced Research Press, 1993.

Chapter Twenty-One: How To Do It

1. Colgan M. **Hormonal Health**. Vancouver: Apple Publishing, 1996.
2. Colgan M. **Essential Fats**. Vancouver: Apple Publishing, in press.
3. Colgan M. **The New Nutrition: Medicine for the Millennium**. Vancouver: Apple Publishing, 1994.
4. Andersson SO, et al. Energy, nutrient intake and prostate cancer risk: a population-based, case-control study in Sweden. **Int J Cancer**, 1996;68:716-722.
5. Patterson BH, Block G, et al. Fruit and vegetables in the American diet: data from the NHANES II Survey. **Am J Public Health**, 1990;80:1443-1449.
6. Colgan M. **Antioxidants: The Real Story**. Vancouver: Apple Publishing, 1998.
7. Colgan M, Colgan LA. **The Flavonoid Revolution**. Vancouver: Apple Publishing, 1997.
8. Thane C, Redd S. Processing of fruits and vegetables: effect on carotenoids. **Nutr and Food Sci**, 1997; March/April:58-65.
9. Oliveria SA, Christos PJ. The epidemiology of physical activity and cancer. **Ann NY Acad Sci**, 1997;833:79-90.

About
Dr. Colgan

Michael Colgan, PhD, CCN, is a renowned lecturer and author of numerous books and articles on nutrition, sports performance and inhibition of aging.

From 1971 to 1982, he was a senior member of the Science Faculty at the University of Auckland, New Zealand. There, he taught in both Human Sciences and the Medical School, while conducting research on human aging and physical performance.

From 1980 to 1982, Dr Colgan was a visiting scholar at Rockefeller University in New York. He has also lectured at Oxford University in England, the University of California in San Diego and the University of Oregon in Washington.

Dr Colgan's professional memberships include the American College of Sports Medicine, the New York Academy of Sciences, the British Society for Nutritional Medicine and the American Academy of Anti-Aging Medicine. He is on the Council of International and American Association of Clinical Nutritionists (the US certification authority for clinical nutritionists), and the Editorial Board of the Journal of Applied Nutrition.

Since 1979, Dr Colgan has been Director of the Colgan Institute.

THE COLGAN INSTITUTE

The Colgan Institute was formed in Auckland, New Zealand, in 1974. In 1982, its head office and laboratory were relocated to San Diego, California.

The Colgan Institute is a consulting, education and research facility, concerned with the effects of nutrition and exercise on sports performance and inhibition of aging.

The Institute has published numerous professional papers, two university texts, five books and over 300 popular articles. It also publishes a monthly magazine, **The Colgan Chronicles**, which has subscribers throughout the world.

In the areas of sports nutrition and longevity, the Institute provides services to major manufacturers and to government in:

- human nutrition research;
- reviews of advances in nutrition;
- analysis of market trends in nutrition; and,
- design of nutritional formulations.

The Institute's clients include, the US National Institute on Aging, the New Zealand Government, and numerous companies including Twinlabs, Weider Health & Fitness, Gull Laboratories, USANA, Nu-Life, Dupont and Digital Equipment.

For the public, the Colgan Institute provides:

- individual nutrition and exercise programs;
- nutrition education programs; and,
- nutrition and training programs for athletes.

DR MICHAEL COLGAN/SPEAKER

Dr Colgan speaks worldwide to sports, medical and corporate organizations, and is frequently invited to speak at a variety of annual conventions. His fast-moving, informative and entertaining lectures on nutrition, aging and athletic performance, draw capacity audiences in the US, Canada, Britain, Australia and New Zealand.

Dr Colgan is a regular speaker at the Arnold Schwarznegger Classic, the Natural Products Expo, the National Nutritional Foods Association Conventions, USANA Conventions, Tegel Foods, Les Mills Gyms, Nu-Life and the International Association of Clinical Nutritionists.

For further information, or to book Dr Colgan to speak at an event, phone 1-760-632-7722, or visit the Colgan Institute web-site at www.colgan-institute.com.

Index

A

Acetyl-l-carnitine 9
Adrenals 9,37
Adverse drug reactions 21
African-American
    prostate disease in 8,14,
    27,28
Albrecht Dr J 62
Alfuzosin 17
Alpha-adrenoceptor antagonists
    alfuzosin 17
    prazosin 17
    tamsulosin 17
    terazosin 17
Alpha-5-reductase 17,20
Alpha-linolenic acid 31
Alpha-Tocopherol, Beta-carotene
    Cancer Prevention
    Study 44
American Cancer Society 13
Anabolic steroids 7,8
Andersson Dr S 24
Androgen
    blocking drugs 9,10,16
    dependent 53
    independent 53,68
Androstenedione 9
Antibiotics 9,72
Antioxidant(s) 41-45

Arrowhead Mills 31
Ascorbic acid 42,80,81

B

Bairati Dr I 27
Basel Prospective Study 44
Barleans 31
Benign prostatic hyperplasia
    (BPH) 1,7-9,12,14-17,20,
    44,48,55,59-62,68,72
Beta-carotene 33-35,42,44,80,81
Beta-sitosterol 55,61

C

Calories 23,24,27,73,80
Canadian Task Force on Periodic
    Health Examinations 13
Cancer
    breast 15,34,37,41,43,48,
    52,66,78
    cell lines 52-53
    endometrium 34,37,41
    prostate 1,2,8-15,24-27,30,
    33,34,37,38,41-45,48,49,
    52,53,55,56,65-69,72,73,78
    skin 51
Carotenoids 33-34

Catalona Dr W 12
Cholecalciferol 52
Citrate 73
Clark Dr L 49
Colgan Institute 5,7,8,26,31,34,
    39,42,45,49,53,57,60,62,
    66,73,75,76,78
    AM/PM Paks 76
    **Prostate Supplement
    Program** 80
Combs Dr G 49
Copper metabolism 73
Cornell University, Ithaca, New
    York 49

D

Daviglus Dr M 42
Degenerative conditions 2
Depression 10,16
DHEA 9
Diadzein 55,56
Dihydrotestosterone (DHT)
    8,16,17,19,53,60,61,65,68
D-alpha-tocopherol 45,80,81
D-alpha-tocopherol succinate
    45,80,81
Dl-alpha-tocopherol 45
Double-bonds 29,30
DU-145 52,53,68

E

East Carolina University School
    of Medicine, Greenville,
    NC 66
Eicosanoids 31
Electroevaporation 16

Ephedrine 9
Epididymis 3,4
Equol 55
Erections 16
Erectile dysfunction 1
Essential Fats 27,29
Essential fats 29,30,77
Essential seco-steroid hormone
    vitamin D 52
Estrogen 61

F

Fair Dr W 27,71
Fat soluble vitamins
    A (retinol) 33
    beta-carotene *(see Beta-
    carotene)*
    D₃ (cholecalciferol) 52,80,
    81
    E (d-alpha-tocopherol)
    45,80,81
    K (phylloquinone)
    41,42,80,81
Finasteride 17,19-22,59-62,68
5-alpha-reductase 60,68
Flax oil 30,31,39,80,81
Flora 31
Food and Nutrition Board of the
    US Institute of Medicine
    75
Food processing 2
Free-PSA 9,11,12
Free radicals 44

G

Garlic 65,66,80

Genistein 55-57
Genistin 56
Getzenberg Dr R 52
Ginseng 9
Glutamine 9
Green tea 67-69,80,81
Gross Dr C 53
Guide to Clinical Preventative
        Services 13

H

Hathcock Dr J 35
Health Professionals Follow-
        up Study 38
HMB 9
Hypericin 9

I

Impotence 5,15,16,62
Immune system 34,41
Incontinence 15
International Union Against
        Cancer 13
Internet
        Guide to Clinical
        Preventive Services 13
        Grateful Med 78
Ion-exchange whey protein
        concentrate 81
Isoflavone(s) 55,56
Israel Dr K 43

J

JAMA 12,21

Journal of the National Cancer
        Institute 38

K

KIC 9
Krebs-Smith Dr S 34
Kyolic aged garlic 66

L

Laser prostatectomy 16
Laval University, Quebec 27
Libido 20
Life Extension Foundation 63
Linoleic acid 29,31
Lipid peroxidation 44
LNCaP 52,53
L-selenomethionine 81
Lycopene 37-39,80,81

M

Marberger Dr M 20
Melatonin 9
Metastasis 43
Metastatic cancer 44,52,53
Mineral ascorbates 42,80,81
Miso 56
Monocytes 34
Multiple vitamin/mineral formula
        42,45,50,54,72,73,75,76,
        80,81

N

National Cancer Institute 34,38,77
National Health Examination
        Surveys 23
Natto 56
Nettle 59,62,63,80,81
Northwestern University
        Medical School, Chicago
        34,42
Nutrition 2,8,10,48,53,78
Nutrition-21 49

O

OKG 9
Olive oil 38
Omega 31
Omega-3 fats 29-31
Omega-6 fats 26,29-31
Ornithine decarboxylase 66-68
Osler Sir William 22

P

Pauling Dr L 42
PC-3 52,53
Penis 3,4
Physicians Health Study 33
Pinto Dr J 65
Polyphenols 68
Prazosin 17
Pregnenolone 9
Preventive Services Task Force 13
Progesterone 61
Prostate
        biopsies 10,12
        cancer 1,2,8,9,11-15,24,
        26,27,30,33,34,37,38,41-
        45,48,49,52,53,55,56,65-
        69,72,73,78
        disease 1-3,5,7,8,12,15,20,
        22,24-27,30,31,33,38,48,
        49,55,56,61,62,72,73,78
        gland 1-5
        infections 9,71,72
        inflammation 1
        overgrowth 3,7,8,12,16,
        19,20,30,37,61,62,67
        surgery 15,16
        transurethral resection 15
        tumor 12,37
Prostatectomy 16
Prostate specific antigen
        (PSA) 9-14,16,19,27,49,53,
        65
Prostatic zinc levels 71
Prostatitis 1,9,12,44,45,61,71,72
Protein Technologies
        International (Supro) 56
Public health policies 2
Pygeum 59-64,80,81
        pygeum africanum 61

R

RDA 47,48,73,75
RDA Committee of the US
        National Academy of
        Sciences 29
Redman Dr C 48
Retinol 33
Rivlin Dr R 65

S

S-allylmercaptocysteine 65,66
Saturated fat 25-27,30
Saw-palmetto 59-64,80,81
Selenium 47-50
Selenomethionine 47-50,80,81
Seminal
    vesicles 3,4
    fluid 72
Sex drive 10
Sexuality 2,3,5,7,61
Sexual potency 5,20
Sigounas Dr G 66
Sloan-Kettering Cancer Center
    New York 25,27,65
Sokeland Dr J 62
Soy
    diet 56
    isoflavones *(see*
    Isoflavones)
    products 55,56
        miso 56
        natto 56
        tofu 56
Spectrum Naturals 31
Sperm 3,5
Stanford University School of
    Medicine, California
    25,53
Steriods 7-9
Steroid hormones 9
    adrenals 9
    pituitary 9
Stinging nettle *(see Nettle)*
Supro soy isolate powder 56,57

T

Tamsulosin 17
Terazosin 17
Testes 3,4,37
Testosterone 8-
    10,16,17,19,53,60,61,65,
    67,68
Tofu 56
Tomatoes 37-39,80
Total PSA 9,11
Transforming growth factor-
    beta 43
Transurethral incision (TUIP) 16
Transurethral needle ablation 16
Transurethral resection of the
    prostate (TURP) 15,16
Tribulus terrestris 9

U

Ultrasound destruction 16
University of Arizona, Tucson
    48,49
University of Munster,
    Germany 62
University of Notre Dame,
    Indiana 56
University of Pittsburgh Cancer
    Institute, Pennsylvania 52
University of Texas, Austin 43
Urethra 2,4,5
Urination 8,17
Urinary
    frequency 3
    function 5
    retention 3

urgency 8
Urologists 1,16
Urology conference, Barcelona,
    Spain 1,17
Urology Dept., Hospital
    University La Fe,
    Valencia, Spain 20
Urtica (*urtica dioica*) 59-64
    stinging nettle 55
US National Cancer Institute
    34,77

V

Vas deferens 3,4
Vitamin A 33
Vitamin C 34,41,42,80,81
Vitamin D 51-54,80,81
Vitamin E 43-46,80,81
Vitamin K 41,42,80,81

W

Wakunaga 66
Walnut oil 30
Western diet 23,25,30,37,38,56
Whittemore Dr A 25

Y

Yohimbe 9

Z

Zinc 75-76,80,81